The CanMEDS Assessment Tools Handbook

An Introductory Guide to Assessment Methods for the CanMEDS Competencies

First Edition

Editors

Glen Bandiera, MD MEd FRCPC
Director, Postgraduate Medical Education
Staff Emergency Physician, Trauma Team Leader
St. Michael's Hospital
Director, FRCP(EM) Residency, University of Toronto

Jonathan Sherbino, MD MEd FRCPC
Department of Emergency Medicine
Hamilton Health Sciences
McMaster University
Clinician Educator, The Royal College of Physicians and Surgeons of Canada

Jason R. Frank, MD MA(Ed) FRCPC
Associate Director, Office of Education
The Royal College of Physicians and Surgeons of Canada
Director of Education, Department of Emergency Medicine, Faculty of Medicine, and
Faculty of Education, University of Ottawa
School of Graduate Studies, Ontario Institute for Studies in Education

The CanMEDS Assessment Tools Handbook
An Introductory Guide to Assessment Methods for the CanMEDS Competencies
First Edition

The Royal College of Physicians and Surgeons of Canada
774 Echo Drive
Ottawa, Ontario K1S 5N8 Canada
Telephone: 1-800-668-3740 or 613-730-8177
Fax: 613-730-8262
Website: royalcollege.ca/canmeds
E-mail: canmeds@royalcollege.ca

Third Printing (Ottawa,ON)

Left cover photo: Wayne Cuddington, Ottawa Citizen. Republished by permission.

ISBN: 9780973915860

How to reference this document:

Bandiera G, J, Sherbino, J R , Frank. The CanMEDS assessment tools handbook. An introductory guide to assessment methods for the CanMEDS competencies. Ottawa: The Royal College of Physicians and Surgeons of Canada; 2006.

Table of contents

Contributors

Glen Bandiera, MD MEd FRCPC
Director, Postgraduate Medical Education
Staff Emergency Physician, Trauma Team Leader
St. Michael's Hospital
Director, FRCP(EM) Residency, University of Toronto

Gary Cole, PhD (Edu)
Senior Research Associate and Manager
Educational Research and Development Unit
Office of Education
The Royal College of Physicians and Surgeons of Canada

Lara Cooke, MD MSc FRCPC
Assistant Professor of Neurology
Assistant Dean of Faculty Development
Faculty of Medicine, University of Calgary

Deepak Dath, MD MEd FRCSC FACS
Program Director
CORE Program in Surgery
McMaster University
St. Joseph's Healthcare, Hamilton

Sue Dojeiji, MD MEd FRCPC
Associate Professor
Director, University of Ottawa Physical Medicine and Rehabilitation Program

Jason R. Frank, MD MA(Ed) FRCPC
Associate Director, Office of Education
The Royal College of Physicians and Surgeons of Canada
Director of Education, Department of Emergency Medicine, Faculty of Medicine and Faculty of Education, University of Ottawa
School of Graduate Studies, Ontario Institute for Studies in Education

Ramona A. Kearney, MD MMEd FRCPC
Associate Professor
Department of Anesthesiology and Pain Medicine
University of Alberta

Erin Keely, MD FRCPC
Acting Head, Division of Endocrinology/Metabolism
Associate Professor of Medicine
Departments of Medicine and Obstetrics/Gynecology
University of Ottawa

George Kovacs, MD ABEM MHPE FRCPC
Associate Professor
Department of Emergency Medicine
Faculty of Medicine
Dalhousie University

Curtis Lee, PhD
Research Associate
Educational Research and Development Unit
Office of Education
The Royal College of Physicians and Surgeons of Canada
Educational Scientist, Department of Emergency Medicine
University of Ottawa

Jocelyn Lockyer, PhD
Associate Dean, Continuing Medical Education and Professional Development
Associate Professor
Department of Community Health Sciences
University of Calgary

Karen Mann, BN MSc PhD
Professor and Director
Division of Medical Education
Dalhousie University

Viren N. Naik, MD MEd FRCPC
Medical Director, Patient Simulation Centre
Assistant Professor
Department of Anesthesia, St. Michael's Hospital
University of Toronto

Ivy Oandasan, MD MHSc CCFP FCFP
Associate Professor and Director
Office of Interprofessional Education
University of Toronto

Derek Puddester, MD FRCPC
Co-Head, Behavioural Neurosciences and Consultation Liaison Team, and
Co-Director, Education, Department of Psychiatry
Children's Hospital of Eastern Ontario
Director, Faculty Wellness Program
Associate Professor, Department of Psychiatry
Faculty of Medicine, University of Ottawa

Saleem Razack, MD
Associate Professor of Pediatrics and Pediatric Residency Program Director
McGill University

Denyse Richardson, MD MEd FRCPC
Assistant Professor, Clinician Educator
Division of Physiatry
Department of Medicine
University of Toronto
Clinician Educator
The Royal College of Physicians and Surgeons of Canada

Jonathan Sherbino, MD MEd FRCPC
Department of Emergency Medicine
Hamilton Health Sciences
McMaster University
Clinician Educator
The Royal College of Physicians and Surgeons of Canada

Sarita Verma, LLB MD CCFP FCFP
Vice Dean
Postgraduate Medical Education
Associate Professor, Department of Family and Community Medicine
Faculty of Medicine, University of Toronto

About this document

One of the most frequently received requests at The Royal College of Physicians and Surgeons of Canada Office of Education is for assessment tools to guide medical educators as they evaluate physician competencies. In response to this need, we have designed this handbook as a resource for medical educators, clinical teachers and all those interested in assessing physician competence using the CanMEDS 2005 Physician Competency Framework.

The handbook draws upon several sources. The tool classification scheme and some of the references are from the CanMEDS Assessment Tools Working Group chaired by Peter Tugwell and colleagues in the 1990s. Supported by a grant from the RCPSC/AMS Endowment Fund for Research in Medical Education, the Working Group assembled a list of tools for assessing the CanMEDS competencies. The CanMEDS office also maintains a bibliography of literature relating to the framework. We searched this database for tools using the terms "evaluation," "assessment" and "competence" and sorted them by CanMEDS Role. The chapter authors of the handbook selected key papers from this source and from the education literature that they believe medical educators will find useful.

This handbook was created for you, and we hope that you will find it of value. This is the first edition, and we expect that updates will be needed as the science of competency-based medical education evolves. We welcome feedback and comments at canmeds@rcpsc.edu and will acknowledge all significant contributions in future editions.

Finally, this document would not have been possible without the extraordinary efforts of the CanMEDS and Faculty Development staff, who skillfully managed the logistics of a multi-authored text. We are grateful to Tammy Hesson, who did an outstanding job coordinating the production of this handbook. We would also like to acknowledge Ginette Bourgeois and Terry Bronstein for their contribution to the production process. We would also like to thank Anne Marie Todkill for her skillful editing and the gordongroup for packaging the content into an accessible format.

The Editors

Introduction

The CanMEDS initiative is a collaborative endeavour to enhance physician competence, professional practice—and, ultimately, patient care. With input from hundreds of Royal College Fellows and staff, family physicians and other medical educators, the initiative has defined a contemporary framework of medical competencies that is aligned with the needs of today's society. Now 11 years old, CanMEDS has been updated as the new *CanMEDS 2005 Framework*.[1]

Implementing the CanMEDS framework requires practical tools for the assessment of physicians' competence in each of their professional roles. Recognizing this need, The Royal College of Physicians and Surgeons of Canada has developed this manual, the *CanMEDS Assessment Tools Handbook*. The handbook is intended to support program directors, rotation coordinators and front-line educators in successfully assessing learner performance in each of the seven CanMEDS Roles.

Three general principles have guided the development of the handbook.

First, the assessment of learners occurs in multiple circumstances over time. Although not every educational setting will lend itself to the assessment of all seven CanMEDS Roles, each Role should be evaluated in a variety of ways specific to relevant settings. Accordingly, the handbook describes several appropriate assessment tools for each CanMEDS Role, enabling educators to choose those tools that best suit their particular program. For example, a program director might use high-fidelity simulation to address several key competencies within the Manager Role. The same program director might also include a short-answer question about quality assurance principles on an in-training written examination, again addressing the Manager Role.

Second, as the Medical Expert Role is central to the CanMEDS framework, direct observation is central to the assessment of performance. Learners can be assessed repeatedly over time by multiple observers as all aspects of medical competence are put into practice. Direct observation, therefore, provides direct insight into actual performance.

Third, we have operationalized the concept of "competence" as a progressive development of abilities. Learners should be assessed at various points in their program to ensure progress along a spectrum of performance and should be provided with guidance for further improvement.

Our intention is that this handbook will serve as a searchable reference for educators seeking quick, practical answers on how to begin to assess specific CanMEDS Roles.

---

[1] Frank JR, editor. *The CanMEDS 2005 physician competency framework. Better standards. Better physicians. Better care.* Ottawa: The Royal College of Physicians and Surgeons of Canada; 2005.

The Handbook

Organized into three sections, the handbook provides both at-a-glance summaries of assessment tools as well as more detailed outlines of their applications, strengths and limitations. Supplementing these brief descriptions, select examples illustrating the tools and approaches described in the handbook will also be posted on the CanMEDS website at http://rcpsc.medical.org/canmeds.

Part 1: Quick reference
This section contains two visual aids. Table 1 provides a rapid outline of the strengths and limitations of common assessment tools. Table 2 presents a matrix that matches appropriate assessment tools to each CanMEDS Role.

Part 2: Overview of contemporary assessment tools
This section provides a more detailed explanation of various assessment tools. Each tool is addressed in a separate chapter, with synopses organized under the following headings:

- Definition
- Advantages
- Disadvantages
- Good for assessing
- Limited ability to assess
- Key points
- References

To ensure that assessment is as objective as possible, tools should be designed to maximize reliability (delivering consistent results in the same situation time after time) and validity (assessing intended knowledge, attitudes, skills or behaviours accepted as legitimate by teachers and learners). It is important, therefore, to tailor the tool to the key competencies being assessed in a given situation and to make assessment items (e.g., short-answer questions, in-training evaluation report statements, checklist items) as explicit and descriptive as possible. An emphasis should be placed on the assessment of concrete, observable learner behaviours or well-defined components of a learner's knowledge base. In developing new tools, users of the handbook are encouraged to consult the references at the end of the chapters for examples of previous work as well as experts in the field of learner assessment.

Part 3: Selected tools for assessing the CanMEDS Roles

This section is based on a detailed literature review specific to each Role. Each chapter focuses on a single CanMEDS Role and on how best to assess learners with respect to that Role. Chapters are organized as follows:

- definition of the CanMEDS Role with associated key competencies
- description and rationale for the best available tools to assess learner performance in that Role
- key literature relating to assessment tools for the specific Role
- other literature relating to the assessment of the specific Role.

The handbook uses typical definitions of assessment tools and reflects the current state of medical education research. Our intent is that, as assessment research advances, updated iterations of this manual will be produced. We trust you will find the handbook useful and invite your feedback.

Glen Bandiera, MD MEd FRCPC
Jonathan Sherbino, MD MEd FRCPC
Jason R. Frank, MD MA(Ed) FRCPC

Part 1: Quick Reference

This section contains two "at-a-glance" visual aids to assist medical educators ascertain the strengths and limitations of common CanMEDS assessment tools (Table 1), and match appropriate assessment tools to each CanMEDS Role (Table 2). These guidelines describe the properties of these types of assessment tools in general. The quality of each specific tool must also be taken into consideration when using these tables.

Table 1: Contemporary Assessment Tools

	Reliability	Validity	Feasibility	Cost	Strengths	Limitations
MCQ	+	+	+	$	Global familiarity Easy to score Extensively researched	Random guessing Difficult to write well Trivialization of content Can overestimate competence
Essay	-	+/-	+/-	$	Assess problem solving Easy to compose	Difficult to score Inefficient Reliability challenges
SAQ	+	+	+	$	Easy to write	Difficult to score
Oral Exam	+/-	+	+/-	-	Assess higher order reasoning Trainee can clarify answers	Time-consuming Examiner cueing Bias issues Standardization issues
OSCE	+	+	-	-	Fidelity Scheduled Assess behaviour in critical events	Deconstructs patient-physician dynamic Limitations of potential simulations Expensive Time-consuming
ITER	-	+	+	$	Assess all domains of competence Flexible Assess behaviour over a period of time Face validity Fidelity	Student characteristics influence assessment of behaviour Poor discriminatory power between domains Reliability issues
MSF	+/-	+	-	$	Assess all domains of competence Interprofessional Many raters	Time intensive May affect patient-physician dynamic Reliability issues Requires proper observer training

	Reliability	Validity	Feasibility	Cost	Strengths	Limitations
Portfolios	-	+/-	-	$	Self-reflection Facilitates remediation Captures performance over time	Time intensive Misrepresentation Adherence / effort
Logbooks	N/A	+/-	+	$	Increases exposure to technical skills Tracking	Assumes repetition equals competence Time consuming Adherence / effort

+ = indicates a characteristic strength of this tool

- = indicates a characteristic weakness of this tool

+/- = varies depending on design of the tool

$ = indicates that the assessment tool is inexpensive. Also, the estimation of assessment tool costs does not include faculty salaries.

Abbreviations:

ITER = In-Training Evaluation Report

MCQ = Multiple Choice Question

OSCE = Objective Structured Clinical Examination

SAQ = Short Answer Question

MSF = Multiple Source Feedback (also referred to as 360 degree evaluation)

[1] Bandiera G, Sherbino J, Frank JR. *The CanMEDS Assessment Tools Handbook. An Introductory Guide to Assessment Methods for the CanMEDS Competencies.* Ottawa: The Royal College of Physicians and Surgeons of Canada; 2006.

Table 2: Key Tools for Assessing the CanMEDS Competencies

	Medical Expert	Communicator	Collaborator	Health Advocate	Manager	Scholar	Professional
1. Written Tests (MCQ, SAQ)	+++	+	++	++	+	++	+
2. Essays	++	+	+	+++	+	+	+
3. Oral Exam	+++	+	+	+	-	-	+
4. Direct Observation and ITER	+++	+++	+++	+++	+++	+++	+++
5. OSCE / SP	+++	+++	+++	++	-	-	+
6. Multi-source Feedback	++	+++	+++	+++	+++	++	+++
7. Portfolio	++	++	+	+++	++	+++	+++
8. Simulations	+++	+	+++	-	++	-	++

+++ = well-suited to assessing many of the Role's key competencies

++ = well-suited to assessing some of the Role's key competencies

\+ = suited to assessing very specific competencies within the Role

\- = not well-suited to the Role

Abbreviations:

ITER = In-Training Evaluation Report

MCQ = Multiple Choice Question

OSCE = Objective Structured Clinical Examination

SAQ = Short Answer Question

SP = Standardized patient

[1] Bandiera G, Sherbino J, Frank JR. *The CanMEDS Assessment Tools Handbook. An Introductory Guide to Assessment Methods for the CanMEDS Competencies.* Ottawa: The Royal College of Physicians and Surgeons of Canada; 2006.

Part 2: Overview of Contemporary Assessment Tools

2.1 Written tests—Constructed-response format (short-answer questions)

Curtis Lee

Definition

The short-answer question (SAQ) format consists of a brief, highly directed question designed to elicit a reliable, constructed response from the learner. Answers usually consist of a few short words or phrases. The model answer key is designed to comprehensively anticipate all correct answers.

Description

SAQs are typically prefaced by a clinical scenario or vignette. The clinical scenario may serve as the basis for several related SAQs.

Marking schemes are well defined for the learner throughout the question to focus the value and structure of the answer. Good SAQs often start with imperatives such as "list" or "name" that define the requirements of the answer. Good SAQs outline the number of items expected in the response and the total possible marks allocated. In addition, the space allotted indicates the expected length of the answer.

Advantages

- tests recall and application of knowledge rather than recognition
- moderate to high reliability
- SAQs tend to have high discrimination indices; this suggests a strong, consistent relation with final assessment outcomes
- simple to administer
- can assess a broad and deep knowledge base
- well-designed questions can be scored objectively
- tend to have a higher face validity than other written formats (candidates answer what they think, rather than selecting from the options provided)
- tend to be easier to create than multiple-choice questions

Disadvantages

- legibility of candidate's handwriting is often problematic
- time-consuming to develop and mark
- difficult to make the answer key comprehensive
- often have a lower face validity than performance-based assessment

Good for assessing

- breadth and depth of factual knowledge in all CanMEDS domains
- clinical application of knowledge and diagnostic reasoning
- problem-solving skills

Limited ability to assess

- behaviour in clinical settings
- written and oral communication skills
- collaborative abilities, such as shared decision-making, team leadership and negotiation
- professionalism, such as integrity, commitment to self-regulated practice and maintenance of personal well-being

Key points

- The development of a model answer key is an essential component of an SAQ.
- When creating SAQs, consider the candidate (Is the question clear and appropriate?) and the marker (Is the model answer key correct and comprehensive? Can responses be scored quickly and objectively?)
- Pilot-test the questions on a sample audience before administering an SAQ examination.

References

http://rcpsc.medical.org/residency/certification/examinerguide/SAQguidelines_e.php

Popham WJ. *Modern educational measurement: practical guidelines for educational leaders*, 3rd ed. Needham (MA): Pearson Education; 2000.

2.2 Written tests—Constructed-response format (essays)

Curtis Lee

Definition

Essays pose questions that require learners to construct an answer based on their knowledge in a written or computer-based format. They require the synthesis and communication of content and often require critical thinking skills such as evaluation, analysis and judgment.

Description

Essay topics may be assigned by the assessor or defined by the learner. *Open-response* essays provide little structure, while *restricted-response* essays provide an outline to improve reliability, including the marker's expectations about content and the amount of time allocated to complete the task. Learners may be allowed to use external resources to research their answer, and they may be able to submit the essay either during a formal exam session or at a later date.

Advantages

- multiple learning objectives can be assessed
- higher-order knowledge can be addressed (e.g., application of factual information)
- simple to develop and administer

Disadvantages

- difficult to score reliably
- learner's approaches to questions are inconsistent and unstandardized
- difficult for markers to avoid the halo or millstone effect (one learner's paper influences the scoring of other essays)
- scoring is time intensive
- markers may be influenced by handwriting, grammar, syntax and spelling
- writing ability and language skills may often be assessed rather than knowledge of content

Good for assessing

- medical expertise (knowledge and attitudes)
- organizational and writing skills
- ability to synthesize information
- written communication
- managerial knowledge base
- approaches to health advocacy
- scholarly knowledge base (e.g., approaches to critical appraisal or teaching)
- professional knowledge base (e.g., applied ethics)

Limited ability to assess

- performance in actual practice
- practice behaviours
- clinical skills and procedures
- collaborative skills (e.g., teamwork and conflict negotiation)

Key points

- After creating an essay question, the assessor should answer the question as part of the development of the answer key. This will allow the assessor to consider the possible range of interpretations the learner may have and to gauge the difficulty of the essay questions and the time necessary to respond to it. Assessors who take this step in developing essay questions typically make modifications to refocus and clarify the question.
- In high-stakes examinations the level of difficulty should be similar for all candidates. Given the challenge of establishing a uniform level of difficulty between essay questions, learners should not be permitted to choose questions from a list.
- It is difficult for markers not to be influenced by the legibility of handwriting and by grammar, syntax and spelling. The use of word processing tools may mitigate these challenges.
- Ideally, marking should be blinded and should be carried out by more than one person. Difficulties in maintaining the learner's anonymity and eliminating bias include the potential to recognize a learner's writing style and the markers' intellectual preferences and interests.

References

Popham WJ. *Modern educational measurement: practical guidelines for educational leaders*. 3rd ed. Needham (MA): Pearson Education Company; 2000.

Violato C, McDougal D, Marini A. *Educational measurement and evaluation*. Dubuque (IA): Kendall/Hunt; 1992.

2.3 Written tests—Selected-response format (multiple-choice, matching, extended matching, pick N and true–false questions)

Curtis Lee

Definition

Selected-response assessment tools consist of a question and a list of options from which the learner must choose the correct answer. All selected-response formats ask the learner to *recognize* the correct answer rather than to recall it without being prompted. Many of these written assessment tools situate the question within a clinical scenario or vignette. Multiple-choice, matching, extended matching, pick N and true–false questions are common tools within this category.

Description

Multiple Choice Questions (MCQs): MCQs consist of an opening question or stem that asks the learner to choose the most correct answer from a list that also includes two to five plausible yet incorrect distractors.

Matching: Learners are given two lists and are asked to match each item in one column to an item in the other column. As a common example, a list of terms in one column is matched with a list of their definitions in the other column.

Extended Matching Questions (EMQs): Learners are given a list of 10 to 20 items and are asked to match them to a series of corresponding responses. An item may be matched to more than one response. For example, learners are given a list of organs and a list of drugs. Learners are asked to match the listed organs to the drugs that affect that organ.

Pick N: An amalgam of MCQs and extended matching, pick N items consist of an opening stem and an instruction to select any given number of correct responses from an extensive list. These questions might ask, for example, for all diagnostic tests or management actions that would be appropriate in a given clinical situation.

True–false: Learners are asked to determine if a given statement is true or false.

Advantages

- can assess diverse content
- questions identical for all learners
- administration is straightforward
- a large number of learners can take the test simultaneously
- marking is objective, simple and comparatively quick
- questions can be banked and reused
- question distribution can reflect weighting of curriculum content
- the legibility of handwriting is not an issue

- can be administered and collated electronically
- item analysis can be performed to determine learner weaknesses and quality of test items

Disadvantages

- assessor cannot determine if correct responses are due to chance
- written tests are language intensive
- low face validity: may not reflect clinical practice or may assess only trivial content
- difficult to create incorrect yet plausible distractors for MCQs
- learners may use deductive reasoning to answer questions, relying on unintentially embedded clues
- question development is time-consuming
- poorly suited for assessment of higher cognitive skills such as synthesis, evaluation and critical thinking

Good for assessing

- knowledge and application of knowledge
- core knowledge in all CanMEDS competencies
- diagnostic reasoning

Limited ability to assess

- communication skills
- collaboration (e.g., teamwork)
- ethical behaviour
- leadership
- organizational skills

Key points

- MCQs can maintain reliability and validity with only three options, likely because two very plausible distractors are used rather than numerous implausible choices.
- Reliability coefficients tend to be high: many questions can be asked quickly and responses have low variance given the limited options.
- Large-scale MCQs can use computer-adaptive semantics that reduce the number of questions. As a learner correctly answers a series of questions, the subsequent questions generated are of increasing difficulty, achieving assessment with fewer questions.
- Keep the main content in the stem rather than in the distracters.
- Avoid the following:
  - assessment of trivial knowledge
  - absolute terms such as “always” or “never”
  - “all the above” or “none of the above” as answer options
  - negative terms such as “not” or ”except” without emphasis

  - Type-K questions that ask learners to choose which combination of a series of statements are correct (e.g., [a] statements 1 and 3; [b] statements 2 and 3; [c] statement 2 only). These are difficult to construct and test logical skills rather than knowledge of content.
- Avoid true–false questions: the probability of guessing the correct answer is high.
- Use matching questions with caution: the formatting of the question may create confusion.
- Extended matching is thought to most closely match clinical practice.
- Learners should be able to pick the correct answer without seeing the distractors.

References

Case SM, Swanson DR. *Constructing written test questions for the basic and clinical sciences.* Philadelphia: National Board of Medical Examiners; 1998. p. 42.

Haladyna TM, Downing SM, Rodriguez MC. A review of multiple-choice item-writing guidelines for classroom assessment. *Appl Meas Educ* 2002;15(3): 309-34.

Wood T, Cole G, Lee C. *Developing multiple choice questions for the RCPSC certification examinations.* Ottawa: The Royal College of Physicians and Surgeons of Canada; 2004. Available: http://rcpsc.medical.org/residency/certification/examinerguide/index.php

2.4 Structured oral examinations (SOEs)

Curtis Lee

Definition

Oral examinations provide an opportunity for an assessor or panel of assessors to pose a series of questions to a learner in order to assess and react to the learner's responses. Oral examinations allow a high level of dynamic interaction between assessor and learner.

Structured oral examinations (SOEs) assess a set number of standardized cases using anticipated probing questions based on the range of expected candidate performance and anchored rating schemata to increase the reliability of the evaluation. SOEs should be used for high-stakes or summative oral assessments. They are usually scored using a predefined, structured template.

Description

Traditionally, oral examinations have consisted of conversations between learners and examiners that potentially cover several general topics or involve an in-depth review and presentation of one case or paper. Although this unstructured approach may result in the assessment of a depth of knowledge and/or the authentic assessment of a particular subject, it is difficult to reproduce the assessment (low reliability) or to generalize success beyond the particular case or topic (case specificity).

Although there are many variations of the oral examination, SOEs typically consist of the review of four to ten cases, each lasting five to fifteen minutes. The entire examination, therefore, lasts about one hour. Each case discussion may include problem-solving, diagnosis, treatment planning, interpretation of results, etc. Role-playing also may be part of a SOE. Ideally, all learners are given the same scenarios, are assessed using the same anchored rating scales, and are given the same reactions to the same responses. Examiners should be trained to focus on the goals of the examination and to refrain from providing the examinee with guiding feedback through verbal cues or body language.

A good SOE will benefit from learner instructions, detailed descriptions of the case scenario (for both learner and assessor), a list of probing questions and responses to anticipated answers, checklists to document candidate's responses, anchored global rating scales and media (e.g., x-ray films, photographs).

Advantages

- tests beyond knowledge base to see how knowledge is applied to a situation
- in formative (learning) assessments, learners can get immediate feedback
- assessor(s) can probe to confirm learner's knowledge or reasoning or to explore competencies to a greater depth

- can be applied to a wide range of competencies and content areas to assess basic knowledge and critical thinking, using a range of hypothetical scenarios
- high face validity: cases can be chosen from typical or critical situations and provided in a realistic manner

Disadvantages

- limited number of cases may lead to content specificity and low reliability
- difficult to standardize
- difficult to implement uniformly by all assessors
- difficult to establish and apply systematic and consistent rating criteria
- difficult to introduce cases identically for each learner
- difficult to avoid giving non-verbal cues
- testing environment may provoke anxiety in learners, leading to poor performance that does not reflect actual competence
- time-consuming: examining ten learners for one hour may require more than one assessor, or more than one working day; a second day of testing may need to be based on different scenarios

Good for assessing

- Medical Expert
  - factual knowledge
  - clinical reasoning skills and problem solving
  - critical thinking (evaluation, synthesis and analysis)
- Communicator
  - interpersonal skills
  - ability to organize information in a clear and logical fashion
- Manager
  - knowledge base (e.g., structure of health care system)
- Health Advocate
  - knowledge of determinants of health
  - knowledge of community services and social supports
- Scholar
  - use of supporting evidence for decisions
- Professional
  - deportment
  - ethical reasoning

Limited ability to assess

- breadth of knowledge
- procedural skills
- physical examination
- actual performance in real situations
- collaboration, teamwork and leadership

Key points

- To promote reliability and validity in SOEs, it is important to invest heavily in the development of the content, case presentations, probing questions and scoring scheme. Improvisation on the part of the assessor decreases the reliability and generalizability of the examination.
- Try to anticipate learner responses and standardized assessment criteria.
- Avoid common rating errors such as the halo effect, regression to the mean, the contract effect, projection, bias, localism and over-generalizations (see the Royal College Guidelines).

References

Guidelines for the conduct of structured oral examinations. Ottawa: The Royal College of Physicians and Surgeons of Canada, 2004.

Finberg L, Lloyd JS. Suggested guidelines for ideal oral examinations. In: Lloyd, JS. *Oral examinations in medical specialty board certification.* American Board of Medical Specialites: Chicago (IL); 1983.

Mancall EL, Bashook PG, editors. *Assessing clinical reasoning: the oral examination and alternative methods.* Evanston (IL): American Board of Medical Specialties; 1995.

2.5 Direct observation

Gary Cole

Definition

In the Royal College model of in-training evaluation, direct observation refers to the ongoing observation, assessment and documentation of actions taken by learners in real clinical settings during their training period. The critical factor that distinguishes direct observation from other forms of assessment is that the learner is observed performing authentic actions that occur naturally as part of daily clinical experience.

Description

Assessed actions can and should relate to any of the CanMEDS Roles and can involve interactions with patients, their relatives, hospital staff, colleagues, students or supervisors. Although any of these individuals could contribute to a learner's assessment (multi-source feedback), direct observation usually implies the observations of an expert (usually the supervisor). Although the setting is always authentic, the arrangement may be more or less formal. In a strictly formal arrangement the learner could be asked to perform a specific task and would be assessed by means of a standardized rating form. In an informal arrangement, no specific planning for the observation would be involved and the assessment would not be recorded on a standardized form. In the latter case, the culmination of observations could inform the completion of a summary In-Training Evaluation Report (ITER) at the conclusion of the educational experience. Ideally, however, learners would be provided with longitudinal feedback to shape their learning.

Advantages

- enables assessment of real-time performance of CanMEDS Roles
- provides opportunities to assess important but infrequent actions
- enables assessment of technical skills that cannot be measured in examinations
- highly useful as formative (learning) assessment, as immediate feedback is usually possible
- assessments from a large number of assessors with a variety of perspectives, are possible
- extreme (good or bad) behaviours in any of the CanMEDS Roles are easily assessed, with important educational consequences
- high face validity

Disadvantages

- when assessment is unstructured and unstandardized, validity and reliability are questionable
- difficult to train observers to be standardized

- different observers might assess different things
- observers might not hold same standard of performance
- little control over the situations observed; resulting behaviours are highly varied
- documentation is sometimes not timely or does not occur at all

Good for assessing

- nearly all key competencies for all CanMEDS Roles
- higher-order behaviours (versus Role knowledge)

Limited ability to assess

- scholarly research competencies
- scholarly lifelong learning

Key points

- Direct observation is one of two methods that assess actual behaviour in the reality of clinical practice.
- Direct observation is particularly appropriate for the assessment of the Communicator, Collaborator and Health Advocate Roles, which are best demonstrated in actual practice. It is an excellent means of assessing higher-order behaviours. When specific tools are used, it is also useful in the assessment of technical skills.
- Direct observation provides good conditions for formative evaluation (immediate feedback).
- Training raters is crucial to the proper use of most assessment tools that use direct observation.
- Input can be obtained from multiple sources, including other health care professionals and patients.
- Although most input is based on unstandardized assessment, the many occasions for observation can cumulatively achieve reasonable validity and reliability.

References

Catton P, Tallett S, Rothman A. A guide to resident assessment for program directors. *Annals RCPSC* 1997;30(7):403-9.

Gray J. Primer on resident evaluation. *Annals RCPSC* 1996;29(2):91-4.

Turnbull J, Gray J, MacFadyen J. Improving in-training evaluation programs. *J Gen Intern Med* 1998;13(May):317-23.

2.6 Objective structured clinical examinations (OSCEs) and objective structured performance-related examinations (OSPREs)

Curtis Lee

Definition

The objective structured clinical examination (OSCE) samples the performance of learners as they rotate through a series of stations representing various clinical scenarios. At each station, learners may encounter a standardized patient, a structured oral examination, visual information (e.g., x-ray films, electrocardiograms), a high- or low-fidelity simulation (e.g., part-task trainer), or a written task. Learners are usually asked to perform a specific skill, to simulate part of a patient encounter, or to answer questions based on the presented material.

The objective structured performance-related examination (OSPRE) is similar to the OSCE, but does not necessarily have a clinical focus.

Description

OSCE circuits typically consist of 8 to 15 stations grouped into a series of rooms and may include one or two rest stations. Learners are usually given 8 to 30 minutes to complete the tasks assigned per room. Learners may have 2 to 5 minutes between stations and may be given information pertaining to the next station during this break. Assessment can be carried out using a standardized checklist, anchored global rating scales, or the evaluation of brief narrative responses.

Advantages

- clinical basis lends high face validity: performance is perceived as more relevant than written assessment
- can focus on specific content areas or skills
- standardizable
- provides direct observation of performance

Disadvantages

- time-consuming to develop
- complex to administer: requires many examiners and many rooms
- only a few content areas can be sampled
- time limitations and testing environment are artificial
- cost-effective only if many learners are assessed

Good for assessing

- history-taking skills
- physical examination skills
- physician–patient communication skills
- diagnostic reasoning, patient management and treatment planning
- knowledge base within a specific context

Limited ability to assess

- complex ethical and professional behaviours
- collaborative interactions
- teaching and research skills
- a large spectrum of knowledge in different areas (given time constraints and limited number of stations)

Key points

- OSCEs are popular for large-scale formative and summative testing. They provide standardized content and testing circumstances, including similar time allocations per station, similar content throughout the examination and similar standardized patient encounters.
- Checklists ensure OSCEs are objective because they optimize consistent marking and fairness, and minimize assessor bias. Checklists—as opposed to global ratings—may yield a better assessment than global ratings. Beware of learners who use the "shotgun" approach, by which they attempt to provide all possible answers in the hope of meeting all checklist criteria.
- Global ratings may be more appropriate in assessing learners with higher levels of expertise. To reduce the level of subjectivity common with global ratings, ensure that ratings scales are anchored for consistent assessment by all assessors.
- Reliability tends to increase with the number of scenarios and stations.

References

Cohen R, Rothman AI, Ross J, Poldre P. Security issues in standardized-patient examinations. *Acad Med* 1993;68(10):S73-S75.

Cohen R, Rothman AI, Ross J, Poldre P. Validating an objective structured clinical examination (OSCE) as a method for selecting foreign medical graduates for a pre-internship program. *Acad Med* 1991;66(9)S67-S69.

Evans J, Morales D, Robb A. *How to run an OSCE: a guide for the beginner.* Toronto: Educating Future Physicians for Ontario (EFPO) Project; 1995.

Hanson M, Russell L, Robb A, Tabak D. *Cross-cultural interviewing: a guide for teaching and evaluation*. Toronto: Faculty of Medicine, University of Toronto: 1996.

Harden R M, Stevenson M, Downie WW, Wilson GM. Assessment of clinical competence using objective structured examination. *BMJ* 1975;1:447-51.

Hodges B, McIlroy JH. Analytic global OSCE ratings are sensitive to level of training. *Med Educ* 2003;37:1012-6.

Hodges B, McNaughton N, Regehr G, Tiberius RG, Hanson M. The challenge of creating new OSCE measures to capture the characteristics of expertise. *Med Educ* 2002;36:742-8.

Hodges B, Regehr G, McNaughton N, Tiberius RG, Hanson M. OSCE checklists do not capture increasing levels of expertise. *Acad Med* 1999;74:1129-34.

Reznick RK, Blackmore DE, Dauphinée WD, Rothman AI, Smee SM. Large-scale high-stakes testing with an OSCE: Report from the Medical Council of Canada. *Acad Med* 1996;S71:19-21.

Rothman AI, Cohen R. Understanding the objective structured clinical examination: issues and options. *Annals RCPSC* 1995;28(5):283-7.

2.7 Standardized patients

Curtis Lee and Jonathan Sherbino

Definition

Standardized patients can be either healthy actors trained to simulate a medical situation or condition or actual patients trained to standardize the presentation of their own condition for assessment purposes. They can be included as part of an Objective Structured Clinical Examination (OSCE) station, as part of an oral examination, or as a stand-alone assessment tool. Although standardized patients have been inserted into clinical practice (e.g., on an outpatient clinic list) without the knowledge of the learner being assessed, this practice raises ethical issues.

As with simulations, standardized patients are not assessment tools in and of themselves. Rather, they provide a means to allow the observation of performance that is then assessed using a standardized checklist, anchored global-rating scale or a brief narrative response.

Description

During an encounter, the standardized patient simulates a real patient presentation using a standardized script. He or she is trained to react to the learner in a standardized way to increase the reliability of the assessment process.

As guided by scenario instructions, direction from the physician assessor or direct interaction with the standardized patient, the learner conducts a clinical evaluation. This may include taking a history, performing a physical assessment, providing a diagnosis, developing a treatment plan, etc.

In addition to the clinical competencies, communication and specific performance skills are often assessed through encounters with standardized patients.

Advantages

- tends to have high face validity because the scenarios are clinically based; performance is perceived as more relevant than written assessment
- allows assessment of focused content areas/skills
- standardized to assess all learners consistently
- involves direct observation of performance

Disadvantages

- time-consuming to train standardized patients and develop scenarios and scripts
- expensive if volunteers are not used
- only a few content areas can be sampled

- pediatric standardized patients require specific debriefing to avoid emotional trauma

Good for assessing

- history-taking (depending on time constraints and scenario design)
- physical examination
- physician–patient communication
- diagnostic reasoning, patient management and treatment planning
- knowledge base within a specific context

Limited ability to assess

- complex ethical and professional behaviours
- genuine collaboration
- critical appraisal and scholar/researcher roles
- a wide spectrum of knowledge in different areas (largely because of time constraints)
- pediatric practice

Key points

- Although real patients are often easier to acquire, learner assessment using real patients tends to result in lower reliability given the difficulty of standardizing the encounter. Maintaining high reliability is important in high-stakes testing such as certification examinations.
- The training of the standardized patient is very important to the development of reliable assessment. Standardized patients must understand the importance of consistent responses and should anticipate probing questions and common interaction. They should know as much as they can about the condition that they are asked to simulate.
- Standardized patients can be trained doctors or other medical professionals. Using these groups greatly reduces the training time required and adds content validity to the assessment.
- Fatigue will be a factor for standardized patients involved in the assessment of a large number of candidates.
- Not all conditions can be simulated (e.g., rheumatoid arthritis, neurological disorders, etc.).
- It is important to ensure that the standardized patient does not have any real physical findings that will distract the learner.

References

Lavallee C. *The examiner's handbook: preparing the standardized patient.* Ottawa: The Royal College of Physicians and Surgeons of Canada; 2006.

Solomon D, Szauter K, Rosebraugh C, Callaway M. Global ratings of student performance in a standardized patient examination: Is the whole more than the sum of the parts? *Adv Health Sci Educ* 2000:5:131-40.

van der Vleuten C, Swanson D. Assessment of clinical skills with standardized patients: state of the art. *Teach Learn Med* 1990;2:58-76.

Wallace J, Rao R, Haslam R. Simulated patients and objective structured clinical examinations: review of their use in medical education. *Adv Psych Treatment* 2002;8:342-50.

Wallace P. Following the threads of an innovation: the history of standardized patients in medical education. *Caduceus* 1997;13(2):5-28.

2.8 Multi-source feedback (360-degree evaluation)

Jocelyn Lockyer

Definition

Multi-source feedback (MSF) is often (erroneously) termed 360-degree evaluation or assessment. This type of evaluation originated in organizational and workplace settings in which supervisors, "direct reports" and peers completed forms to gather information, appraise conduct and provide feedback. MSF uses specific instruments designed to gather data about particular behaviours or professional constructs (e.g., professionalism and communication skills) of the learner. In educational settings, observers may include physicians (e.g., resident peers, supervising physicians and medical students), allied health professionals (e.g., nurses, pharmacists and psychologists), patients and family members. A self-assessment is frequently included. The questionnaires may be the same or different for each of the assessor groups. Feedback is provided in aggregate form for each source. MSF can be used to provide formative and summative assessments, and identify learners in difficulty.

Description

MSF usually includes feedback solicited from two or more sources, potentially including the learner. Feedback is typically provided by completing a questionnaire-based tool consisting of 10–40 items that is designed to assess clinical behaviours that can be observed and remediated. MSF can supplement traditional sources of assessment (e.g., examinations and preceptor observations) by providing input from people who do not normally have a hierarchal responsibility for providing feedback, yet may have a different perspective on actual learner performance. Finally, MSF encourages reflection and promotes development of a self-improvement plan.

Advantages

- assesses behaviours
- reliability is obtained by virtue of the number of assessors providing feedback
- can be used for formative purposes to guide self-improvement in specific areas or to identify learners at risk
- supplements other assessments
- makes values and behaviours explicit
- adaptable to changing environments and assessment needs
- facilitates development of reflection and insight through comparison of source feedback with self assessment.
- aggregate data may inform curriculum strengths and weaknesses
- assesses some behaviours that are difficult for traditional methods to assess

Disadvantages

- survey items and constructs of interest must be meticulously designed to achieve a valid tool that appropriately assesses behaviour
- requires an appropriate sample of assessors for reliability. Generalizability studies can determine the appropriate sample size (e.g., 8–10 peers, 8–10 health professionals, 25 or more patients, depending on the number of survey items)
- requires a stable infrastructure for survey distribution, data collation and reporting
- requires ongoing, significant input from assessors
- language barriers may influence patient participation
- stimuli are daily, real events that are random and different for every observer; lack of standardization creates challenges in data interpretation and reliability analyses
- feedback is provided by people who do not have a hierarchical relationship with the learner; resultant feedback, although anonymous, may be unexpected and influence team relationships

Good for assessing

- interpersonal communication
- professionalism
- interprofessional team work abilities
- advocacy for patients, addressing determinants of health

Limited ability to assess

- knowledge base and technical skills (best left to expert observers)

Key points

- MSF is a questionnaire-based tool designed to assess observable behaviours that are amenable to remediation.
- Sufficient items and observers are required to provide reliable information to the learner.
- Considerable infrastructure is required.

References

Archer JC, Norcini J, Davies HA. Use of SPRAT for peer review of paediatricians in training. *BMJ* 2005;330:1251-3.

Johnson D, Cujec B. Comparison of self, nurse, and physician assessment of residents rotating through an intensive care unit. *Crit Care Med* 1998;26(11):1811-6.

Joshi R, Ling FW, Jaeger J. Assessment of a 360-degree instrument to evaluate residents' competency in interpersonal and communication skills. *Acad Med* 2004;79:458-63.

Violato C, Lockyer J, Fidler H. The assessment of pediatricians by a regulatory authority, *Pediatrics* 2006;117:796-802

Useful websites

www.par-program.org
The College of Physicians and Surgeons of Alberta
This website provides copies of the questionnaires used in Alberta to assess family physicians, surgeons, anesthesiologists, internists, pediatricians, psychiatrists, episodic care physicians (e.g., emergency physicians, locum physicians, hospitalists) and radiologists, along with background information about the program and the feedback report. Although it is designed to provide quality improvement data for practising physicians, the information contained on the website, as well as the examples, will be helpful in developing MSF assessment tools.

http://www.mmc.nhs.uk/pages/foundation/foundation-learning-portfolio
Foundations Program (United Kingdom)
The Foundations Program encompasses PGY 1 and PGY 2 trainees in the UK. As part of the development program for the trainee, two types of MSF are used. Mini-Pat is based on the domains of Good Medical Practice (comparable to CanMEDS competencies). The other MSF tool assesses team-based behaviours.

2.9 Portfolios and logbooks

Jason R. Frank, Karen Mann and Erin Keely

Definitions

Portfolios provide a flexible, multifaceted means of collecting evidence of the achievement of competence over time. Logbooks are structured instruments for documenting that a learning activity has taken place.

Description

Clinical faculty may be familiar with portfolios in the context of teaching dossiers that are used in applications for academic promotion. However, portfolios as well as logbooks have many definitions and applications in the medical and educational literature. Growing interest in competency-based education and in new concepts of competence that go beyond the Medical Expert Role is increasing the popularity of these assessment tools.

Portfolios are an extremely flexible educational technology that can be adapted to multiple purposes, settings and kinds of learners. Both portfolios and logbooks can be used to collect evidence that learning has taken place. We define logbooks as those tools that are used to track the incidence of educationally relevant activities, such as the number of procedures performed (e.g., a list of appendectomies). They tend to be highly structured, giving little or no opportunity for learner input or reflection. At the other end of the spectrum are unstructured tools that give learners autonomy in deciding what represents their work and provide ample opportunity for reflection. An artist's diary would be an example of this. In the middle lies the kind of portfolio that most contemporary medical programs would find useful: deliberately designed, structured, defining domains of activity and markers of competencies, but capturing supervisor observations on achievement of competence and learner reflections on learning over time.

In this way, portfolios are really an "instrument of instruments," or a collection of assessment tools. Their components may include logbooks, multi-source feedback instruments, continuous quality improvement projects, learning diaries, encounter cards, essays, rating scales, etc. When designing a portfolio for assessment, it is important to be clear not only on its purpose, but also on the role of the learner in collecting the material, the degree of reflection desired, the medium (e.g., paper or online), and on how expectations and standards will be set.

Advantages

- high authenticity
- flexible, allowing multiple ways to demonstrate achievement
- can be learner-centred, reflecting individual goals and interests

- can facilitate dialogue between learner and teacher, especially when learner is involved in setting criteria for achievement and quality of evidence
- involve learner in creating, gathering and assessing evidence
- longitudinal rather than cross-sectional, allowing for demonstration of growth
- stimulate self-directed learning
- provide opportunities to reflect on learning and plan new goals
- can include assessments from a variety of sources (e.g., peers and patients)
- can have a positive educational impact
- can be employed across the spectrum of medical education, from medical school to residency to continuing professional development
- analysis of records can be used for program evaluation or accreditation (e.g., procedure logbooks)

Disadvantages

- only as useful as the component parts: breadth, validity and reliability depend on the instruments used to gather data and can be time-consuming to create and to assess
- requires appropriate design and development of evaluation criteria
- requires review and input by the teacher
- may be difficult to standardize
- depending on the design, may be resource-intensive
- learner compliance may be poor if the portfolio has low perceived utility or relevance
- effective use may require a culture change in many medical settings

Good for assessing

- complex performance and integrative competencies in all CanMEDS Roles
- documentation of procedural activities
- various aspects of the Communicator Role (written, oral, interpersonal)
- portfolios—may be the strongest method to assess Scholar competencies of lifelong learning, research and teaching
- demonstrates evidence of collaboration and teamwork; good for assessing performance in authentic situations
- excellent for providing ongoing formative assessment

Limited ability to assess

- Medical Expert Role
- situations in which all learners must demonstrate the same competency in a standardized way
- situations where summative decisions are being taken and high reliability is required

Key points

- Portfolios offer the opportunity to assess complex competencies that can be demonstrated in different ways by different persons under different conditions.
- They offer a high potential for learning through assessment and an opportunity to develop skills that will be needed for lifelong maintenance of competence.
- Portfolios require careful design and development, with particular regard to purpose, criteria for and evidence of achievement. As yet, they are most effective for formative evaluation and documenting progress.
- The literature suggests that successful portfolio use is associated with supervisor support and regular, periodic review.
- Although portfolios may promote learner reflection, they do not ensure that it will occur.
- There must be support for the use of portfolios in the setting in which they will be used, by both learners and teachers.

References

Carraccio C, Englander R. Evaluating competence using a portfolio: a literature review and web-based application to the ACGME competencies. *Teach Learn Med* 2004;16(4):381-7.

Chisholm CD, Croskerry P. A case study in medical error: the use of the portfolio entry. *Acad Emerg Med* 2004;11(4):388-92.

Davies H, Khera N, Stroobant J. Portfolios, appraisal revalidation, and all that: a user's guide for consultants. *Arch Dis Child* 2005;90:165-70.

Davis MH, Friedman Ben-David M, Harden RM, Howie P, Ker J, McGhee C, et al. Portfolio assessment in medical students' final examinations. *Med Teach* 2001;23:357-66

Doezema D, McLaughlin S, Sklar DP. An approach to fulfilling the systems-based practice competency requirement. *Acad Emerg Med* 2002;9(11):1355-9.

Driessen EW, van Tartwijk J, Vermunt JD, van der Vleuten CP. Use of portfolios in early undergraduate medical training. *Med Teach* 2003;25:18-23.

Friedman B, David M, Davis MH, Harden RM, Howie PW, Ker J, Pippard MJ. AMEE Medical Education Guide no. 24: Portfolios as a method of student assessment. *Med Teach* 2001;23:535-51.

Fung MF, Walker M, Fung KF, Temple L, Lajoie F, Bellmare G, et al. An internet-based learning portfolio in resident education: The KOALA multicentre programme. *Med Educ* 2000;34(6):474-9.

Grant A, Dornan TL. What is a learning portfolio? *Diabet Med* 2001;18(Suppl. 1):1-4.

Hays RB. Reflecting on learning portfolios. *Med Educ* 2004;38(8):801-3.

Holmboe ES, Rodak W, Mills G, McFarlane MJ, Schultz HJ. Outcomes-based evaluation of resident education: Creating systems and structured portfolios. *Am J Med* 2006;119(8):708-14.

Jarvis RM, O'Sullivan PS, McClain T, Clardy JA. Can one portfolio measure the six ACGME general competencies? *Acad Psychiatry* 2004;28:190-6.

Lonka K, Slotte V, Halttunen M, Kurki T, Tiitinen A, Vaara L, et al. Portfolios as a learning tool in obstetrics and gynecology undergraduate training. *Med. Educ.* 2001;35(12):1125-30.

O'Sullivan P, Green C. Portfolios: Possibilities for addressing emergency medicine resident competencies. *Acad Emerg Med* 2002;9:1305-9.

O'Sullivan PS, Reckase MD, McClain T, Savidge MA, Clardy JA. Demonstration of portfolios to assess competency of residents. *Adv Health Sci Ed* 2004;9:309-323

Pinsky L, Fryer-Edwards K. Diving for PERLS. Working and performance portfolios for evaluation and reflection on learning. *J Gen Intern Med* 2004;19:582-7.

Rees CE, Sheard CE. The reliability of assessment criteria for undergraduate medical students' communication skills portfolios: The Nottingham experience. *Med Educ* 2004;38:138-44.

Roberts C, Newble DI, O'Rourek AJ. 2002. Portfolio-based assessments in medical education: Are they valid and reliable for summative purposes? *Med Educ* 2002;36(10):899-900.

2.10 Simulation-based assessment

Viren N. Naik and Glen Bandiera

Definition

Simulation is the artificial recreation of a clinical environment or circumstance for the purpose of allowing a learner to undertake a specific task in a controlled manner that presents no risk to patients. Simulation can recreate many clinical settings with a degree of realism, allowing educators to observe how individuals and teams may perform in the "real world." Simulation is particularly useful in assessing learner performance of a complete procedure, or in crisis situations that might not commonly be encountered or managed independently during a finite residency.

Description

Simulation encompasses a broad spectrum of instructional and research tools. For example, standardized patients are a form of simulation discussed elsewhere in this handbook. Part-task trainers are models made of plastic and latex that simulate body areas with anatomical correctness to allow trainees to practise specific technical procedures. These models can incorporate components of "virtual reality." For example, high-fidelity full-body simulation uses computer-driven mannequins to recreate patient care in floor beds, operating rooms, intensive care units and emergency rooms. These mannequins mimic physical findings (e.g., heart and breath sounds), but more importantly, their physiologic parameters respond to interventions by participants, such as the administration of oxygen, drugs, fluids and chest compressions.

Rather than being an assessment tool in and of itself, simulation is a venue in which other more traditional tools can be applied. Measuring performance with the use of simulation can achieve high validity and reliability by applying specific criteria in controlled conditions. Direct observation is a commonly used assessment modality in simulation, and can be carried out using checklists, global ratings or multiple scales for specific behaviours. Alternatively, learners could be asked to produce, for inclusion in a portfolio, a brief report on their experience and a prescription for future work. Both formative and summative evaluations are possible with simulation. Procedural skills are best evaluated on part-task trainers. Checklists break down a particular procedure into several key items that can be scored as done correctly or incorrectly. General domains common to all technical procedures can be assessed with global-rating scales, including ordinal Likert scales. The management of dynamic simulated emergencies requires both medical expertise and behavioural skills to make decisions and lead a team effectively. There are several global ratings systems for crisis management in the literature with established content and construct validity.

Advantages

- measures performance of entire procedure from start to finish
- measures performance in emergencies
- measures individual or team performance
- provides a standardized and controlled testing environment
- face validity is potentially high
- formative and summative assessments are possible
- allows learners to practise high-risk procedures in a safe environment and to encounter rare scenarios

Disadvantages

- increasing fidelity dramatically increases cost
- resource intensive (space, equipment and personnel)
- requires considerable commitment of faculty time
- technical challenges

Good for assessing

- Medical Expert
  - entire procedures
  - emergency management scenarios
- Communication
  - patient and family interaction during and after scenarios
- Collaboration
  - teamwork
  - interprofessional competencies
  - conflict resolution
- Manager
  - crisis resource management
  - leadership behaviours
- Professional
  - self-control
  - ethical decision-making
  - self-assessment
  - respectful interactions with team

Limited ability to assess

- Health Advocate Role
- Scholar Role

Key points

- Ensure learners are familiarized with simulated environment and limitations prior to formative and summative evaluations.
- Faculty development with respect to simulator-based assessment procedures is essential before undertaking this form of assessment.
- Experienced simulator operators are essential for standardization.
- This form of assessment is often stressful for learners; debriefing is required.
- Validated methods and scale designs are available in the literature to guide evaluations and debriefing.

References

Ali J, Gana TJ, Howard M. Trauma mannequin assessment of management skills of surgical residents after advanced trauma life support training. *J Surg Res* 2000;93:197-200.

Bond WF, Spillane L. The use of simulation for emergency medicine resident assessment. *Acad Emerg Med* 2002;9(11):1295-9.

Fletcher G, Flin R, McGeorge P, Glavin R, Maran N, et al. Anaesthetists' Non-Technical Skills (ANTS): Evaluation of a behavioural marker system. *Brit J Anaesth* 2003;90(5):580-8.

Gaba DM, Howard SK, Flanagan B, Smith BE, Fish KJ, Botney R. Assessment of clinical performance during simulated crises using both technical and behavioural ratings. *Anesthesia* 1998;89(1):8-18.

Martin JA, Regehr G, Reznick R, MacRae H, Murnaghan J, Hutchison C, et al. Objective structured assessment of technical skill (OSATS) for surgical residents. *Brit J Surg* 1997;84(2):273-8.

Regehr G, MacRae H, Reznick RK, Szalay D. Comparing the psychometric properties of checklists and global rating scales for assessing performance on an OSCE-format examination. *Acad Med* 1998;73(9):993-7.

Reznick R, Regehr G, MacRae H, Martin J, McCulloch W. Testing technical skill via an innovative "bench station" examination. *Am J Surg* 1997;173(3):226-30.

Savoldelli GL, Naik VN, Joo HS, Houston PL, Graham M, Yee B, et al. Evaluation of patient simulator performance as an adjunct to the oral examination for senior anesthesia residents. *Anesthesiology* 2006;104(3):475-81.

Weller JM, Bloch M, Young S, Maze M, Oyesola S, Wyner J, et al. Evaluation of high fidelity patient simulator in assessment of performance of anaesthetists. *Brit J Anaesth* 2003:90(1):43-7.

2.11 Encounter cards

Jason R. Frank, Curtis Lee and Glen Bandiera

Definition

Encounter cards are a type of in-training tool characterized by direct observations that are documented after brief encounters between the supervisor and the learner in a clinical setting. They are also known as:

- daily evaluation cards (DECs)
- daily encounter cards (DECs)
- daily operative cards (DOCs)
- daily shift cards
- daily teaching evaluation cards (DTECs)
- teaching encounter cards (TECs)
- interaction cards
- feedback forms

Description

Encounter cards and their variants are a method of direct assessment that helps the assessor to capture observations of clinical competence from brief encounters with learners. They are especially useful when a single learner is working with multiple assessors during a clinical rotation. Encounter cards are therefore increasingly popular in emergency medicine, critical care, anesthesiology and some surgical disciplines.

Typically, the cards are completed and discussed collaboratively at the end of a discrete period of clinical work, such as a shift in the emergency department, intensive care unit, ambulatory clinic, operating room, etc. By implementing a system that involves learners and assessors in a standardized manner immediately after the observed clinical duties, documented formative feedback can be timely, frequent and grounded on examples from the day. Encounter cards thus improve the validity and reliability of in-training assessment and provide opportunities to review rotation expectations and to discuss achievements, strengths and areas for improvement.

When CanMEDS based rotation objectives are used to develop the items included, encounter cards are useful for competency-based assessment. Assessments can be recorded qualitatively (as comments), quantitatively (as Likert scores), or both. Scales should be anchored by descriptive terms that reflect behaviours specific to the clinical environment. In addition, providing observers with training on what behaviours can be reflected on each encounter card scale can increase reliability and validity of the resulting assessment. Encounter card systems designed in this way can be used to inform summative end-of-rotation assessments and to document strengths and weaknesses for promotion decisions, and can be fed into a database to track performance over time.

Finally, encounter cards can also be used to facilitate the more frequent assessment of teaching. By this method, learners complete an encounter card designed to capture teaching competence for that brief period (e.g., a day in the operating room or a shift in the emergency department).

Advantages

- provide a regular opportunity to reinforce expectations for a rotation
- create a forum for frequent, timely, grounded and formative feedback
- facilitate input from multiple assessors on multiple occasions over a rotation
- document directly observed performance
- enable performance to be tracked over time
- may contribute to summative In-Training Evaluation Reports (ITERs)
- when clinical cases are recorded, they provide a method for tracking clinical exposure for each learner and for the rotation as a whole

Disadvantages

- to work well, evaluation cards require assessors and learners to frequently find time to discuss assessment
- requiring cards at the end of every encounter may lead to "assessment fatigue" and "gaming" of the forms
- faculty development is required to prepare assessors to use the cards effectively and provide useful feedback
- cards are typically submitted at the end of the shift, when learners and assessors may be tired
- performance ratings may be consistently high or absent, depending on the cases seen during the shift and thus may not represent true ability
- a single observation period may not provide an opportunity to assess performance in every domain of the encounter card
- faculty tend to skew observations to the positive end of the spectrum; even with well-designed scoring systems, the "halo" and "millstone" effect as well as central tendency can skew assessment

Good for assessing

Nearly every CanMEDS key competency can be assessed, depending on the structure of the encounter card, the setting and the discipline. This would include:

- Medical Expert: clinical decision-making, histories, physicals, therapies and integration of the other Roles
- Communicator: abilities with patients and families; charting
- Collaborator: team interactions and conflict management
- Manager: use of resources, efficiency, leadership and practice management
- Health Advocate: advocacy for individual patients and the ability to recognize systemic issues

- Scholar: teaching ability, critical appraisal and ability to apply evidence, educational strategies for filling in knowledge
- Professional: behaviours relating to professionalism

Limited ability to assess

- comprehensive breadth of knowledge, skills and attitudes.
- Scholar – research abilities.
- Professional – ability to work within a profession framework and sustainable practice

Key points

- Encounter cards are a type of direct assessment that can be designed to reflect any or all the CanMEDS Roles.
- They facilitate timely, frequent, grounded feedback.
- They provide a system for multiple assessors to assess a single learner.
- They can enhance the validity and reliability of in-training assessment.
- They can contribute to summative assessment reports.
- They can track the case mix of learners.

References

Al-Jarallah K, Moussa MA, Shebab D, Adella N. Use of interaction cards to evaluate clinical performance. *Med Teach* 2005; 27(4):269-74.

Bennet AJ, Goldenhar LM, Standford K. Utilization of a formative evaluation card in a psychiatry clerkship. *Acad Psychiatry* 2006;30(4):319-24.

Brennan BG, Norman GR. Use of encounter cards for evaluation of residents in obstetrics. *Acad Med* 1997;72(10 Suppl. 1):S433-4.

Colletti M. Difficulty with negative feedback: face-to-face evaluation of junior medical student clinical performance results in grade inflation. *J Surg Res* 2000;90(1):82-7.

Greenberg LW. Medical students' perceptions of feedback in a busy ambulatory setting: a descriptive study using a clinical encounter card. *South Med J* 2004;97(12):1174-8.

Kernan WN, Holmboe E, O'Connor PG. Assessing the teaching behaviours of ambulatory care preceptors. *Acad Med* 2004;79(11):1088-94.

Kim S, Kogan JR, Bellini LM, Shea JA. A randomized-controlled study of encounter cards to improve oral case presentation skills of medical students. *J Gen Intern Med* 2005;20(8):743-7.

Paukert JL, Richards ML, Olney C. An encounter card system for increasing feedback to students. *Am J Surg* 2002;283(3):300-4.

Part 3: Selected Tools for Assessing the CanMEDS Competencies

3.1 Medical Expert: knowledge-based competencies

Glen Bandiera

Definition

As Medical Experts, physicians integrate all of the CanMEDS Roles, applying medical knowledge, clinical skills and professional attitudes in their provision of patient-centred care. Medical Expert is the central physician Role in the CanMEDS framework.

Key competencies

Physicians are able to …

1. Function effectively as consultants, integrating all of the CanMEDS Roles to provide optimal, ethical and patient-centred medical care;
2. Establish and maintain clinical knowledge, skills and attitudes appropriate to their practice;
3. Perform a complete and appropriate assessment of a patient;
4. Use preventive and therapeutic interventions effectively;
5. Demonstrate proficient and appropriate use of procedural skills, both diagnostic and therapeutic;
6. Seek appropriate consultation from other health professionals, recognizing the limits of their expertise.

Overview

The Medical Expert Role is central to overall physician competence and, as such, is the Role most familiar to those who assess medical learners. This Role can be manifested both in what learners know and in what they do. Attitudes, while affecting eventual performance, are harder to assess but are usually manifested in a learner's behaviour. Competence in this Role involves obtaining a body of factual knowledge deemed relevant, current and appropriately comprehensive, as well as problem-solving through the application of this knowledge. Finally, the Medical Expert Role implies an ability to coordinate one's performance of the other six CanMEDS Roles to maximize the effectiveness of clinical practice for each patient and the community served.

This chapter does not address the assessment of procedural competency in the Medical Expert Role; this topic is specifically addressed in the next chapter.

Preferred tools

1. Direct observation and in-training evaluation reports
Most Medical Expert key competencies are amenable to assessment through direct observation. Observation of clinical care allows learners to demonstrate their application of knowledge and higher-order thinking. Questioning during patient encounters or teaching sessions (such as ward rounds) permits direct observation of factual knowledge. The indications, complications and steps pertaining to procedures can be evaluated. Finally, a learner's ability to integrate all CanMEDS Roles into clinical care is best assessed during the day-to-day clinical care of patients. Ideally, ITERs will be completed on the basis of repeated observations over time, with each observation resulting in feedback to the learner to foster the development of competence.

Much has been written about the design of ITERs and the ability of observers to be objective in their assessments of multiple dimensions of performance. Well-designed ITERs are specific to the behaviours of interest, have clear descriptors for each level of performance and promote the use of the entire assessment scale. However, most ITER-based systems still have problems with recall bias, the halo effect and central tendency. Training assessors will reduce but not eliminate these concerns.

2. Written examinations
Written tests have long been central to the assessment of a learner's knowledge base. They can test factual knowledge and, when properly designed, higher-order problem-solving and diagnostic reasoning. Multiple-choice questions (MCQs) and short-answer questions (SAQs) are preferred over essays and other forms of narrative response in view of their higher reliability and more objective marking parameters. Although properly designed MCQs and SAQs are hard to develop, they can be highly reliable and thus are used on many certification examinations. Written tests appeal to learners because they serially gauge the developing knowledge base and help prepare learners for a component of the certification examination experience.

Written examinations cannot assess actual clinical performance; rather, they assess the foundational knowledge on which performance is based.

3. Oral examinations
Oral examinations are time- and resource-intensive. They are, however, one of the best methods for assessing a learner's ability to apply knowledge to clinical scenarios. Although written tests are efficient at assessing pure factual knowledge, oral examinations are appropriate for assessing integration of facts, formation and prioritization of differential diagnoses, development of management plans and difficult decision-making. Oral examinations allow learners to interact with the assessor and demonstrate their ability to thoroughly assess and manage patient problems.

To maximize reliability, exam material must be standardized, and oral examiners need to be trained in the delivery of information and the assessment of responses. Without these steps, oral examinations can have marginal reliability as a result of assessor variability, loss of focus on intended subject areas, and impaired learner performance due to inappropriate examiner disclosure or questioning.

4. Objective structured clinical examinations (OSCEs)
OSCEs are effective assessment tools for a variety of clinical domains. However, since they are resource- and time-intensive they should be used only for scenarios in which other assessment tools are less appropriate. OSCEs are useful for testing the application of knowledge in specific clinical settings that are high-risk, difficult to observe in practice, or rare.

OSCEs are intended to provide multiple "samples" of a learner's ability; however, they suffer from limited generalizability in that performance in a given clinical scenario does not necessarily reflect performance in all related areas. OSCE stations require global-rating scales, checklists or standardized patient feedback to generate assessment data.

5. Simulation
Simulation involves a spectrum of assessment tools, ranging from standardized patients to partial-task trainers to high-fidelity, computer-driven mannequins. All of these tools can be adapted to assess knowledge, procedural skills, clinical reasoning, etc. Simulation can be used alone or as a component of OSCE stations. Used alone, simulation is useful for testing, potentially with a high degree of realism, the application of knowledge in specific clinical settings. Learners are tasked with carrying out a clinical activity designed to assess a specific domain of knowledge. Because of the resource-intensive nature of simulation, it is best reserved for multifaceted tasks involving difficult decisions and clinical reasoning. Application of the fundamental principles of leadership, teamwork and collaboration can also be assessed.

Key literature

1. Jouriles N, Burdick W, Hobgood C. Clinical assessment in emergency medicine. *Acad Emerg Med* 2002;9:1289–94.

Tool type
Various

Study design
Descriptive review

Study population
Emergency medicine residents

Comments

This review was carried out by a subcommittee of American program directors to describe the most appropriate methods for assessing clinical skills. They focus on direct observation and simulated patients as the most appropriate methods and offer suggestions as to how to include them in a residency program.

2. Coderre SP, Harasym P, Mandin H, Fick G. The impact of two multiple-choice question formats on the problem-solving strategies used by novices and experts. *BMC Med Educ* 2004;4:23.

Tool type

Written examination: multiple-choice questions

Study design

Experimental single cohort

Study population

Gastroenterology learners and experts

Comments

The authors listened to physicians at various levels of training and practice while they verbally worked through an MCQ examination to determine how they would approach different types of multiple-choice questions. This study lends insight on how a multiple-choice question can test higher-order thinking and how to properly design such questions.

3. Holmboe ES. Faculty and the observation of trainees' clinical skills: problems and opportunities. *Acad Med* 2004;79(1):16-22.

Tool type

Direct observation

Study design

Review

Study population

Medical students and residents

Comments

This excellent review article examines the disadvantages and some of the inherent biases of direct observation and discusses challenges in improving this method. Solutions are offered to help increase the degree to which the assessment of actual behaviour is reflected in written reports.

4. Gray JD. Global rating scales in residency education. *Acad Med* 1996;71(1 Suppl):S55-63.

Tool type
Direct observation, ITERs

Study design
Review article

Study population
Medical residents

Comments
This is an excellent review of the design and use of rating scales to assess resident performance. It describes the principles of scale design and ways to introduce rating scales to maximize the accuracy of the resulting assessments.

5. Wass V, Van der Vluten C, Shatzer J, Jones R. Assessment of clinical competence. *Lancet* 2001;357:945-9.

Tool type
Written examinations, direct observation, standardized patients, OSCEs

Study design
Review

Study population
Medical residents

Comments
This review article makes the case for multi-modal assessment and explains the ideal roles for various assessment methods in an overall resident assessment program.

Other literature

Bandiera G, Morrison LJ, and Regehr G. Predictive validity of the global assessment form used in a final-year undergraduate rotation in emergency medicine. *Acad Emerg Med* 2002;9(9):889-95.

Day RP et al. Evaluation of resident performance in an outpatient internal medicine clinic using standardized patients. *J Gen Intern Med* 1993;8(4):193-8.

Estes NC, Conlee L S., DeBord-Smith A, Smith E, Whittaker, Jr LD, Rossi TR. The value of using naijve observers to assess resident ACGME competencies. *Curr Surg* 2004;61(6):629-35.

Norman GR et al. Measuring physicians' performances by using simulated patients. *J Med Edu* 1985;60(12):925-34.

Prislin MD et al. Use of an objective structured clinical examination in evaluating student performance. *Fam Med* 1998;30(5):338-44.

Rethans JJ et al. Competence and performance: two different concepts in the assessment of quality of medical care. *Fam Pract* 1990;7(3):168-74.

Sargeant J, Mann K, Ferrier S. Exploring family physicians' reactions to multisource feedback: perceptions of credibility and usefulness. *Med Edu* 2005;39(5):497-504.

Shapiro MJ, Kobayashi L, Morchi R. High-fidelity medical simulation and its role in evaluation advanced cardiac life support (ACLS) skills. *Acad Emerg Med* 2003;10(5):488.

Stillman PL, Swanson DB. Ensuring the clinical competence of medical school graduates through standardized patients. *Arch Intern Med* 1987;147(6):1049-52.

Turnbull J et al. Clinical work sampling: A new approach to the problem of in-training evaluation. *J Gen Intern Med* 2000;15(8): 556-61.

Vu NV et al. Standardized (simulated) patients' accuracy in recording clinical performance checklist items. *Med Educ* 1992;26(2):99-104.

Rethans JJ, Norcini JJ, Baron-Maldonado M, Balckmore D, et al. The relationships between competence and performance: implications for assessing practice performance. *Med Educ* 2002;36:901-9.

3.2 Medical Expert: procedural skills competencies

George Kovacs

Definition

As Medical Experts, physicians integrate all of the CanMEDS Roles, applying medical knowledge, clinical skills and professional attitudes in their provision of patient-centred care. Medical Expert is the central physician Role in the CanMEDS framework.

Key competencies

Physicians are able to ...

1. Function effectively as consultants, integrating all of the CanMEDS Roles to provide optimal, ethical and patient-centred medical care;
2. Establish and maintain clinical knowledge, skills and attitudes appropriate to their practice;
3. Perform a complete and appropriate assessment of a patient;
4. Use preventive and therapeutic interventions effectively;
5. *Demonstrate proficient and appropriate use of procedural skills, both diagnostic and therapeutic;*
6. Seek appropriate consultation from other health professionals, recognizing the limits of their expertise.

Overview

Procedural skills involve the mental and motor activities required to execute a manual task. Procedural skill competence requires both safe technical performance and appropriate knowledge for decision-making in the preparation, performance and post-performance phases of the procedure.

Formative assessment of a procedure should involve more than simply a decision about whether or not a learner can do the procedure safely. Assessment of a procedure at its completion (e.g., assessing a sutured laceration), although useful, leaves out important assessment points that address questions of process. For example, task efficiency has been shown to correlate with psychomotor skill and may be represented by the number of hand movements and the time to completion. The experienced clinician will make significantly fewer fine-motor movements and will take less time than a novice to successfully complete a procedural task.

Ideally, procedural skill assessment tools should be fixed, objective outcome measures and should be reliable, valid and feasible.

Preferred tools

1. Simulation

Limited opportunities for clinical exposure and ethical concerns have contributed to the development of simulation to both learn and assess procedural skills. Although validation of these newer and often expensive technologies remains slow, simulation is rapidly gaining acceptance as a means to assess procedural skills. The value of simulation is that learners can practise procedures in a standardized environment that poses no risk to patients. Serial assessment can document learner progression from safe performance to mastery, including an appropriate knowledge base and the insight to recognize when the limits of one's technical abilities necessitates consultation with a colleague.

Whether it be related to specific skills on part-task trainers or complete procedures demonstrated in the course of a high-fidelity, computer-driven mannequin simulation, assessment in the simulation environment will require the use of standardized checklists or global assessment scores.

2. Direct observation and In-Training Evaluation Reports (ITERs)

The performance of procedures in the course of clinical activities can be assessed using ITERs. Assessment may be quantitative (How many did the learner do?) or qualitative (How good was the performance?). However, this form of assessment for procedural skills is potentially limited by the halo effect, central tendency and recall bias. For example, assessment of specific procedures would require a distinct item on the ITER for every procedure likely to be encountered on a rotation, creating a laborious task for the assessor. Alternatively, condensing all procedures into one or two broad statements neglects the fact that learners may be good at some procedures and poor at others. One way to address this would be to include general principles of procedures (obtaining proper consent, adhering to sterile technique, etc.) as specific items and to use a separate section to list procedures properly done and those in need of improvement.

It is possible to add specific observational assessment tools to a clinical environment to complement the ITER. For example, global rating scales have been developed, validated and shown to be reliable tools for assessing performance in the operating room.

3. Logbooks

Logbooks provide important, necessary, quantitative procedural skill data. Without these data it is difficult to know whether learners are being exposed to an adequate range and volume of "core" procedures. Although volume alone should never define competence, it has been clearly linked to procedural outcomes. An accepted methodology for predefining minimum needs in terms of procedural volume has not been clearly established. Recently, the cumulative sum (CUSUM) statistical method has been developed as a technique to address this issue. CUSUM can correlate the number of technical procedures with competent performance. When used in association with logbooks, CUSUM is able to rapidly detect changes in performance of technical procedures associated with adverse outcomes.

Procedural notes and, more specifically, operative notes do provide detailed descriptions that require "visualization" of a specific procedure from start to finish. There is minimal literature on the validity and reliability of using operative notes for the assessment of procedural skills.

3. Objective structured clinical examinations (OSCEs)
OSCEs often include task procedure assessment. For example, the Objective Structured Assessment of Technical Skills (OSATS) has been used and validated in the postgraduate surgical setting. It is essentially a technical skill OSCE comprising model "bench" tasks. Also, the McGill Inanimate System for Training and Evaluation of Laparoscopic Skills (MISTELS) has been widely used to assess component laparoscopy skills. Both tools have literature supporting their reliability, construct and predictive validity.

Key literature

1. Ahlberg G, Hultcrantz R, Jaramillo E, Lindblom A, Arvidsson D. Virtual reality colonoscopy simulation: a compulsory practice for the future colonoscopist? *Endoscopy* 2005;37(12):1198-204.

Tool type
Simulation, global assessment form (satisfaction, time, outcomes)

Study design
Randomized interventional trial

Study population
Endoscopy residents and staff

Comments
Virtual-reality simulators have evolved rapidly as trainers for endoscopy. This study is an example of this tool, demonstrating predictive validity and skill transfer for colonoscopy.

2. Van Rij AM, McDonald JR, Pettigrew RA, Putterill MJ, Reddy CK, Wright JJ. CUSUM as an aid to early assessment of the surgical trainee. *Br J Surg* 1995;82(11):1500-3.

Tool type
Direct observation: CUSUM forms

Study design
Prospective observational

Study population
Surgical residents

Comments
This study demonstrated that standardized, validated instruments can be applied to direct observation for early detection of residents in difficulty.

---

3. Datta V, Bann S, Beard J, Mandalia M, Darzi A. Comparison of bench test evaluations of surgical skill with live operating performance assessments. *J Am Coll Surg* 2004;199:603–6.

Tool type
Simulation with direct observation and validated assessment form

Study design
Prospective observational comparison of assessment techniques

Study population
Staff and resident surgeons

Comments
This study compares simulated observation with "real-world" observation and demonstrates both an effective use of a validated scale and the validity of simulation-based assessments.

---

4. Fried GM, Feldman LS, Vassiliou MC, Fraser SA, Stanbridge D, Ghitulescu G, Andrew CG. Proving the value of simulation in laparoscopic surgery. *Ann Surg* 2004;240(3):518-25.

Tool type
Simulation with validated direct observation form

Study design
Prospective observational

Study population
Surgical residents and staff

Comments
MISTELS has been validated as a tool to both teach and assess laparoscopic skills.

5. Hayden SR, Panacek EA. Procedural competency in emergency medicine: the current range of resident experience. *Acad Emerg Med* 1999;6(7):728-35.

Tool type
Logbooks and portfolios

Study design
Observational cohort

Study population
Emergency medicine residents

Comments
This study demonstrates that there is program variation related to procedure exposure. "Adequate" exposure is yet to be defined but is a consideration that should not be ignored.

6. Olsen JC, Gurr DE, Hughes M. Video analysis of emergency medicine residents performing rapid-sequence intubations. *J Emerg Med* 2000;8(4):469–72.

Tool type
Direct observation, videotaping

Study design
Prospective observational

Study population
Emergency medicine residents

Comments
This study reviews an innovative way to provide feedback on actual clinical performance of high-stakes, relatively rare events.

7. Reznick R, Regehr G, MacRae H, Martin J, McCulloch W. Testing technical skill via an innovative "bench station" examination. *Am J Surg* 1997;173(3):226-30.

Tool type
OSCE with checklists and global ratings

Study design
Prospective interventional

Study population
Surgery residents

Comments

This study contributed to the literature validating bench simulation as a means of assessing surgical skills.

Other literature

Ahlberg G, Hultcrantz R, Jaramillo E, Lindblom A, Arvidsson D. Virtual reality colonoscopy simulation: a compulsory practice for the future colonoscopist? *Endoscopy* 2005;37(12):1198-204.

Bann S, Davis IM, Moorthy K, Munz Y, Hernandez J, Khan M, Datta V, Darzi A. The reliability of multiple objective measures of surgery and the role of human performance. *Am J Surg* 2005;189(6):747-52.

Birkmeyer JD, Stukel TA, Siewers AE, Goodney PP, Wennberg DE, Lucas FL. Surgeon volume and operative mortality in the United States. *N Engl J Med* 2003;349(22):2117-27.

Boyd KB, Olivier J, Salameh JR. Surgical residents' perception of simulation training. *Am Surg* 2006;72(6):521-4.

Bullock G, Kovacs G, Macdonald K, Story BA. Evaluating procedural skills competence: inter-rater reliability of expert and non-expert observers. *Acad Med* 1999;74(1):76-8.

Chou B, Handa VL. Simulators and virtual reality in surgical education. *Obstet Gynecol Clin North Am* 2006;33(2):283-96, viii-ix.

Datta V, Bann S, Mandalia M, Darzi A. The surgical efficiency score: a feasible, reliable, and valid method of skills assessment. *Am J Surg* 2006;192(3):372-8.

Feldman LS, Hagarty SE, Ghitulescu G, Stanbridge D, Fried GM. Relationship between objective assessment of technical skills and subjective in-training evaluations in surgical residents. *J Am Coll Surg* 2004;198(1):105-10.

Kobayashi L, Shapiro MJ, Sucov A, Woolard R, Boss RM 3rd, Dunbar J, Sciamacco R, Karpik K, Jay G. Portable advanced medical simulation for new emergency department testing and orientation. *Acad Emerg Med* 2006;13(6):691-5.

Kovacs G, Bullock G, Ackroyd-Stolarz S, Cain E, Petrie D. A randomized controlled trial on the effect of educational interventions in promoting airway management skill maintenance. *Ann Emerg Med* 2000;36(4):301-9.

Kovacs G. Procedural skills in medicine: linking theory to practice. *J Emerg Med* 1997;15(3):387-91.

MacDonald J, Williams RG, Rogers DA. Self-assessment in simulation-based surgical skills training. *Am J Surg* 2003;185(4):319-22.

Miller GE. The assessment of clinical skills/competence/performance. *Acad Med* 1990;65(9 Suppl):S63-7

Moorthy K, Munz Y, Adams S, Pandey V, Darzi A; Imperial College – St. Mary's Hospital Simulation Group. Self-assessment of performance among surgical trainees during simulated procedures in a simulated operating theater. *Am J Surg* 2006;192(1):114-8.

Mulcaster JT, Mills J, Hung OR, MacQuarrie K, Law JA, Pytka S, Imrie D, Field C. Laryngoscopic intubation: learning and performance. *Anesthesiology* 2003;98(1):23-7.

Murray DJ, Boulet JR, Kras JF, McAllister JD, Cox TE. A simulation-based acute skills performance assessment for anesthesia training. *Anesth Analg* 2005;101(4):1127-34.

Munz Y, Moorthy K, Bann S, Shah J, Ivanova S, Darzi SA. Ceiling effect in technical skills of surgical residents. *Am J Surg* 2004;188(3):294-300.

Nestel D, Kneebone R, Black S. Simulated patients and the development of procedural and operative skills. *Med Teach* 2006; 28(4):390-1.

Regehr G, MacRae H, Reznick RK, Szalay D. Comparing the psychometric properties of checklists and global rating scales for assessing performance on an OSCE-format examination. *Acad Med* 1998;73(9):993-7.

Reznick RK, Regehr G, Yee G, Rothman A, Blackmore D, Dauphinee D. Process-rating forms versus task-specific checklists in an OSCE for medical licensure. Medical Council of Canada. *Acad Med* 1998;73(10 Suppl):S97-9.

3.3 Communicator

Sue Dojeiji and Lara Cooke

Definition

As Communicators, physicians effectively facilitate the physician–patient relationship and the dynamic exchanges that occur before, during and after the medical encounter.

Key competencies

Physicians are able to ...

1. Develop rapport, trust and ethical therapeutic relationships with patients and families;
2. Accurately elicit and synthesize relevant information and perspectives of patients and families, colleagues and other professionals;
3. Accurately convey relevant information and explanations to patients and families, colleagues, and other professionals;
4. Develop a common understanding on issues, problems and plans with patients and families, colleagues and other professionals to develop a shared plan of care;
5. Convey effective oral and written information about a medical encounter.

Overview

Effective communication is a core domain of medical competence. As reviewed by Kurtz et al (2005), physicians with effective verbal, non-verbal, and written communication abilities foster therapeutic physician-patient relationships, and strengthen rapport with families and other health professionals. Effective communication enhances patient outcomes, adherence, satisfaction and safety. Competence in the Communicator Role is therefore essential for all physicians and must be taught, reinforced, and assessed throughout the continuum of medical education. Although communication skills may be learned, they can also deteriorate over time if they are not reiterated and evaluated on an ongoing basis.

Assessing the Communicator Role poses some unique challenges. There is a common perception that communication skills are more subjective than objective or more truly a reflection of "natural gifts" than of observable and measurable skills. However, the literature clearly demonstrates that communication skills can be taught, learned and measured in a reliable and structured manner.

Arguably, the most valid means of assessing any competency is to directly observe the trainee performing in his or her usual work environment and to assess a pre-determined set of relevant and identifiable behaviours. The reality of residency training is that this is not always possible. Therefore, different assessment tools may be necessary in different settings.

Preferred tools

1. Direct obervation and In-Training Evaluation Reports (ITERs)
Direct observation of trainees' communication skills remains the most valid method of assessing communication abilities. Assessment through direct observation is best achieved by using a skills-based, reliable and valid assessment tool that will allow any clinical supervisor to objectively evaluate learners' communication skills during their training. Detailed checklists can be used to specifically address communications skills in a given practice situation. Examples of such checklists include the Calgary Cambridge Observation Guide, the Kalamazoo Checklist and the SEGUE framework. ITERs are also well suited to assessing communication abilities longitudinally in actual practice. ITERs can be created to meet the individual needs of each training program, thus reflecting the essential communication skills required within that specialty.

2. Objective structured clinical examinations (OSCEs) and standardized patients
OSCEs and standardized patients are commonly used to assess communication skills and allow assessment under relatively controlled conditions. OSCEs also allow the practice and assessment of difficult, infrequent or sensitive communication tasks, which may not always be possible in real practice. Learners can be observed taking a history or counselling standardized patients in OSCE stations. Feedback can be provided by observers or by the standardized patients themselves if they are properly trained.

3. Multi-source feedback
Multi-source feedback is increasingly being used to assess communication abilities. Multiple raters, including patients, allied health care professionals and peers can provide valuable data to guide further learning.

4. Portfolios and logbooks
These tools can track activities involving ongoing learning of communication competencies, including written communication (e.g., consultation letters and discharge summaries). More importantly, portfolios promote reflection on practice and may be effective tools for self-directed enhancement in this competency.

Key literature

1. Boon H, Stewart M. Patient-physician communication assessment instruments: 1986 to 1996 in review. *Patient Educ Couns* 1998;35(3):161-76.

Tool type
Various

Study design
Systematic review

Study population
Mixed (undergraduate, postgraduate, in-practice)

Comments
This is an excellent systematic review; however, the search strategy ends at 1996.

---

2. Duffy FD, Gordon GH, Whelan G, Cole-Kelly K, Frankel R, Buffone N, et al. Assessing competence in communication and interpersonal skills: the Kalamazoo II report. *Acad Med* 2004;79(6):495-507.

Tool type
Various

Study design
Consensus statement

Study population
Mixed (undergraduate, postgraduate)

Comments
This excellent consensus statement provides a comprehensive overview of both communication skills assessment tools and measurement scales.

---

3. Hobgood CD, Riviello RJ, Jouriles N, Hamilton G. Assessment of communication and interpersonal skills competencies. *Acad Emerg Med* 2002;9(11):1257-69.

Tool type
Direct observation and standardized patients

Study design
Consensus statement

Study population
Postgraduate, emergency medicine

Comments

This article provides a consensus list of desired communication behaviours. It also supplies a preferential, annotated list of assessment tools and associated measurement scales.

---

4. Ram P, Grol R, Rethans JJ, Schouten B, van der Vleuten C, Kester A. Assessment of general practitioners by video observation of communicative and medical performance in daily practice: issues of validity, reliability and feasibility. *Med Educ* 1999;33(6):447-54.

Tool type

Direct observation

Study design

Cross-sectional

Study population

General practitioners

Comments

This study determined the psychometric properties of video-recorded direct observation by a physician assessor. Study participants reported that the video camera did not interfere with their practice.

---

5. Keely E, Myers K, Dojeiji S. Can written communication skills be tested in an objective structured clinical examination format? *Acad Med* 2002;77(1):82-6.

Tool type

Objective structured clinical examination

Study design

Cross-sectional

Study population

Postgraduate, internal medicine

Comments

This study demonstrated that a validated rating scale and global assessment scores were effective in the assessment of written communication skills (consultation letters).

Other literature

Baldwin PJ, Paisley AM, Brown SP. Consultant surgeons' opinion of the skills required of basic surgical trainees. *Brit J Surg* 1999;86(8):1078-82.

Booth K, Maguire P, Hillier VF. Measurement of communication skills in cancer care: myth or reality? *J Adv Nurs* 1999;30(5):1073-9.

Boulet JR et al. Assessing the comparability of standardized patient and physician evaluations of clinical skills. *Adv Health Sci Educ Theory Pract* 2002;7(2):85-97.

Buller MK, Buller DB. Physicians' communication style and patient satisfaction. *J Health Soc Behav* 1987;28:375-88.

Butterfield PS, Mazzaferri EL. A new rating form for used by nurses in assessing residents' humanistic behavior. *J Gen Intern Med* 1991;6(2):155-61.

Campion P, Foulkes R, Tate P. Patient centredness in the MRCGP video examination: analysis of large cohort. *BMJ* 2002;325:691-2.

Carnay SL, Mitchell KR. Satisfaction with medical students' clinical skills. *J Med Educ* 1986;61(5):374-9.

Carney SL, Mitchell KR. Satisfaction of patients with medical student's clinical skills. *J Med Educ* 1986:61(5):374-9.

Cassata DM, Conroe RM, Clements PW. A program for enhancing medical interviewing using videotape feedback in the family practice residency. *J Fam Pract* 1977;4(4):673-7.

Chalabian J, Dunnington G. Standardized patients: a new method to assess the clinical skills of physicians. *Best Pract Benchmarking Healthc* 1997;2(4):174-7.

Chur-Hansen A. The self-evaluation of medical communication skills. *HERDSA* 2001;20(1):71-79.

Colliver JA et al. Effects of examinee gender, standardized patient gender, and their interaction on standardized patients' ratings of examinees' interpersonal and communication skills. *Acad Med* 1993;68(2):153-7.

Colliver JA et al. Relationship between clinical competence and interpersonal and communication skills in standardized-patient assessment. *Acad Med* 1999;74(3):271-4.

Cowan DH, Laidlaw JC. A strategy to improve communication between health care professionals and people living with cancer. I. Improvement of teaching and assessment of doctor–patient communication in Canadian medical schools. *J Cancer Educ* 1993;8(2):109-17.

Cowan DH et al. Consensus statement from the workshop on the teaching and assessment of communication skills in Canadian medical schools. *CMAJ* 1992;147(8):1149-52.

Dale J et al. Primary care consultation skills training: implementing a new training program for senior house officers in an accident and emergency department. *Med Educ* 1997;31(4):243-9.

Daniel AE, Burn RJ, Horarik S. Patients' complaints about medical practice. *Med J Aust* 1999;170(12):598-602.

de Haes JC et al. Assessment of medical students' communicative behaviour and attitudes: estimating the reliability of the use of the Amsterdam attitudes and communication scale through generalizability coefficients. *Patient Educ Couns* 2001;45(1):35-42.

Des Marchais JE, Jean P, Castonguay LG. Training psychiatrists and family doctors in evaluating interpersonal skills. *Med Educ* 1990;24(4):376-81.

Dibben MR, Morris SE, Lean ME. Situational trust and co-operative partnerships between physicians and their patients: a theoretical explanation transferable from business practice. *QJM* 2000;93(1):55-61.

Duberman TL. Assessing the critical behavioral competencies of outstanding managed care primary care physicians. *Manag Care Interface* 1999;12(3):76-80.

Duffy FD, Gordon GH, Whelan G, Cole-Kelly K, Frankel R, Buffone N, et al. Assessing competence in communication and interpersonal skills: the Kalamazoo II report. *Acad Med* 2004;79(6):495-507.

Eggly S et al. An assessment of residents' competence in the delivery of bad news to patients. *Acad Med* 1997;72(5):397-9.

Elwyn G et al. Measuring the involvement of patients in shared decision-making: a systematic review of instruments. *Patient Educ Couns* 2001;43(1):5-22.

Fallowfield L et al. Efficacy of a cancer research UK communication skills training model for oncologists: a randomized controlled trial. *Lancet* 2002;359(9307): 650-6.

Feletti GI, Carney SL. Evaluating patients' satisfaction with medical students' interviewing skills. *Med Educ* 1984;18(1):15-20.

Finlay IG, Stott NC, Kinnersley P. The assessment of communication skills in palliative medicine: a comparison of the scores of examiners and simulated patients. *Med Educ* 1995;29(6):424-9.

Gallagher TJ, Hartung PJ, Gregory SW. Assessment of a measure of relational communication for doctor–patient interactions. *Patient Educ Couns* 2001;45(3):211-8.

Girgis A, Sanson-Fisher RW, McCarthy WH. Communicating with patients: surgeons perceptions of their skills and need for training. *Aust N Z J Surg* 1997;67(11):775-80.

Girgis A, Sanson-Fisher RW, Walsh RA. Preventive and other interactional skills of general practitioners, surgeons, and physicians: perceived competence and endorsement of postgraduate training. *Prev Med* 2001;32(1):73-81.

Haddad S et al. Patient perception of quality following a visit to a doctor in a primary care unit. *Fam Pract* 2000;17(1):21-29.

Hargie O et al. A survey of communication skills training in UK schools of medicine: present practices and prospective proposals. *Med Educ* 1998;32(1):25-34.

Henbest RJ, Stewart MA. Patient-centredness in the consultation. 1: A method for measurement. *Fam Pract* 1989:6(4):249-53.

Hobgood CD Riviello RJ, Jouriles N, Hamilton G. Assessment of communication and interpersonal skills competencies. *Acad Emerg Med* 2002;9(11):1257-69.

Hobma SO et al. Setting a standard for performance assessment of doctor-patient communication in general practice. *Med Educ* 38 2004;(12):1244-52.

Humphris GM, Kaney S. The Liverpool brief assessment system for communication skills in the making of doctors. *Adv Health Sci Educ Theory Pract* 2001;6(1):69-80.

Jarski RW et al. A comparison of four empathy instruments in simulated patient–medical student interactions. *J Med Educ* 1985;60(7):545-51.

Johnson D, Cujec B. Comparison of self, nurse, and physician assessment of residents rotating through an intensive care unit. *Crit Care Med* 1998;26(11):1811-6.

Jouriles NJ, Emerman CL, Cydulka RK. Direct observation for assessing emergency medicine core competencies: interpersonal skills. *Acad Emerg Med* 2002;9(11):1338-41.

Keely E, Myers K, Dojeiji S. Can written communication skills be tested in an objective structured clinical examination format? Acad Med 2002;77(1):82-6.

Keely E, Dojeiji S, Myers K. Writing effective consultation letters: 12 tips for teachers. *Med Teach* 2002;24(6):585-9.

Keen AJ, Klein S, Alexander DA. Assessing the communication skills of doctors in training: reliability and sources of error. *Adv Health Sci Educ Theory Pract.* 2003;8(1):5-16.

Kisch AI, Reeder LG. Client evaluation of physician performance. *J Health Soc Behav* 1969;10:51-8.

Kosower E, Inkelis S, Seidel J. Telephone TALK : a teaching/assessment tool for medical training. *J Biocommun* 1996;23(1):22-6.

Kosower E et al. Evaluating telephone TALK. *J Biocommun* 1996;23(1):27-31.

Kurtz SM. Doctor–patient communication: principles and practices. *Can J Neurol Sci* 2002;29(Suppl 2):S23-9.

Kurtz S, Silverman J, Draper J. *Teaching and learning communication skills in Medicine*. 2nd ed. Radcliffe Publishing, Oxford UK; 2005.

Lang F et al. Faculty development in communication skills instruction: insights from a longitudinal program with "real-time feedback." *Acad Med* 2000;75(12):1222-8.

Makoul G. Essential elements of communication in medical encounters: the Kalamazoo consensus statement. *Acad Med* 2001;76(4):390-3.

Makoul G, Schofield T. Communication teaching and assessment in medical education: an international consensus statement. Netherlands Institute of Primary Health Care. *Patient Educ Couns* 1999;37(2):191-5.

Makoul G, Altman M. Early assessment of medical students' clinical skills. *Acad Med* 2002;77(11):1156.

Makoul G. The interplay between education and research about patient–provider communication. *Patient Educ Couns* 2003;50(1):79-84.

Marcotte DB, Held JP. A conceptual model for attitude assessment in all areas of medical education. *Med Educ* 1978;53(4):310-4.

Martin D et al. Using videotaped benchmarks to improve the self-assessment ability of family practice residents. *Acad Med* 1998;73(11):1201-6.

Merrill JM et al. Measuring "humanism" in medical residents. *South Med J* 1986;79(2):141-4.

Meuleman JR, Harward MP. Assessing medical interview performance. Effect of interns' gender and month of training. *Arch Intern Med* 1992;152(8):1677-80.

Miller SJ, Hope T, Talbot DC. The development of a structured rating schedule (the BAS) to assess skills in breaking bad news. *Br J Cancer* 1999;80(5-6):792-800.

Moulton D. "Patient navigators" newsiest members of NS health care team. *CMAJ* 2002;167(3):295.

Mullan PB, Stross JK. Sensitivity to patients' psychosocial concerns: relationships among ratings by primary care and traditional internal medicine house officers and patient self-assessments. *Soc Sci Med* 1990;31(12):1337-45.

Nunez AE. Transforming cultural competence into cross-cultural efficacy in women's health education. *Acad Med* 2000;75(11):1071-80.

O'Keefe M. Should parents assess the interpersonal skills of doctors who treat their children? A literature review. *J Paed Child Health* 2001;37(6):531-8.

O'Keefe M et al. Medical student interviewing: a randomized trial of patient-centredness and clinical competence. *Fam Pract* 2003;20(2):213-9.

Oandasan I et al. Developing competency-assessment tools to measure the family physician's ability to respond to the needs of the community. *Acad Med* 2001;76(10):S80-S1.

Page GG et al. Physician-assessment and physician-enhancement programs in Canada. *CMAJ* 1995;153(12):1723-8.

Pell I et al. Development and preliminary evaluation of a clinical guidance program for the decision about prophylactic oophorectomy in women undergoing a hysterectomy. *Qual Saf Health Care* 2002;11(1):32-9.

Quest TE et al. The use of standardized patients within a procedural competency model to teach death disclosure. *Acad Emerg Med* 2002;9(11):1326-33.

Ram P, Grol R, Rethans JJ, Schouten B, van der Vleuten C, Kester A. Assessment of general practitioners by video observation of communicative and medical performance in daily practice: issues of validity, reliability and feasibility. *Med Educ* 1999;33(6):447-54.

Ramsey PG et al. Use of peer ratings to evaluate physician performance. *JAMA* 1993;269(13):1655-60.

Redelmeier DA et al. Problems for clinical judgment: 2. Obtaining a reliable past medical history. *CMAJ* 2001;164(6):809-13.

Reisner E et al. A model for the assessment of students' physician–patient interaction skills on the surgical clerkship. Am J Surg 1991;162(3):271-3.

Roter D et al. The effects of a continuing medical education program in interpersonal communication skills on doctor practice and patient satisfaction in Trinidad and Tobago. *Med Educ* 1998;32(2):181-9.

Roter DL et al. An evaluation of residency training in interviewing skills and the psychosocial domain of medical practice. *J Gen Intern Med* 1990;5:347-54.

Roth CS, Watson KV, Harris IB. A communication assessment and skill-building exercise (CASE) for first-year residents. *Acad Med* 2002;77(7):746-7.

Russell ML, Insull W, Jr , Probstfield JL. Examination of medical professions for counseling on medication adherence. *Am J Med* 1985;78(2):277-82.

Sanson-Fisher RW et al. Training medical practitioners in information transfer skills: the new challenge. *Med Educ* 1991;25(4):322-33.

Scott J et al. The impact of training in problem-based interviewing on the detection and management of psychological problems presenting in primary care. *Br J Gen Pract* 1999;49(443):441-5.

Segall A, Burnett M. Patient evaluation of physician role performance. *Soc Sci Med* 1980;14A:269-78.

Sleight P. Teaching communication skills: part of medical education? *J Hum Hypertens* 1995;9(1):67-9.

Snell L et al. A review of the evaluation of clinical teaching: new perspectives and challenges. *Med Educ* 2000;34(10):862-70.

Soh KB. Job analysis, appraisal and performance assessments of a surgeon: a multifaceted approach. *Singapore Med J* 1998;39(4):180-5.

Stein REK et al. Severity of Illness: concepts and measurements. *Lancet* 1987;1506-9.

Stewart M et al. Evidence on patient-doctor communication. *Cancer Prev Control* 1999;3(1):25-30.

Stilwell NA, Reisine S. Using patient-instructors to teach and evaluate interviewing skills. *J Dent Educ* 1992;56(2):118-22.

Stott NC et al. Innovation in clinical method: diabetes care and negotiating skills. *Fam Pract* 1995;12(4):413-8.

Tate P et al. Assessing physicians' interpersonal skills via videotaped encounters: a new approach for the Royal College of General Practitioners Membership Examination. *J Health Commun* 1999;4(2):143-52.

Taylor KL, Chudley AE. Meeting the needs of future physicians: a core curriculum initiative for postgraduate medical education at a Canadian university. *Med Educ* 2001;35(10):973-82.

Thomson AN. Consumer assessment of interview skills in a family practice certification examination. *Fam Med* 1993;25(1):41-4.

Usherwood T. Subjective and behavioural evaluation of the teaching of patient interview kills. *Med Educ* 1993;27(1):41-7.

Weaver MJ et al. A questionnaire for patients' evaluations of their physicians' humanistic behaviors. *J Gen Intern Med* 1993;8(3):135-9.

Woolliscroft JO et al. Evaluating the medical history: observation versus write-up review. *J Med Educ* 1984;59(1):19-23.

Woolliscroft JO et al. Resident-patient interactions: the humanistic qualities of internal medicine residents assessed by patients, attending physicians, program supervisors, and nurses. *Acad Med* 1994;69(3):216-24.

3.4 Collaborator

Ivy Oandasan and Denyse Richardson

Definition

As Collaborators, physicians effectively work within a health care team to achieve optimal patient care.

Key competencies

Physicians are able to ...

1. Participate effectively and appropriately in an interprofessional health care team;
2. Effectively work with other health professionals to prevent, negotiate, and resolve interprofessional conflict.

Overview

A collaborative practice approach involving interprofessional teams of health care providers and offering comprehensive and coordinated health care services has been proposed as a fundamental way to enhance the Canadian health care system (Kirby,[1] Romanow,[2] Health Council of Canada[3]).The 2003 First Ministers' Accord on Health Care Renewal identified the importance of changing the way health care professionals are educated. The CanMEDS Collaborator Role addresses this call. Physicians who are competent collaborators will gain the knowledge, skills, attitudes and behaviours to work effectively with other health professionals and thus enhance the delivery of patient-centred care.

It has been reported that health professionals engaged in interprofessional learning activities gain an increased understanding of the roles, responsibilities, strengths and limitations of other professions. They develop attitudes of mutual respect and willingness to collaborate with other members of the health care team. Evidence has shown that effective teamwork in health care can enhance clinical care outcomes, increase provider satisfaction, improve patient safety and augment organizational efficiencies.

[1] Kirby MLJ. *The health of Canadians: the federal role. Final report*. Ottawa: Standing Senate Committee on Social Affairs, Science and Technology, 2002.

[2] Romanow R. *Building on values: the future of health care in Canada*. Saskatoon: Commission on the Future of Health Care in Canada; 2002.

[3] Health Council of Canada. *Modernizing the management of health human resources in Canada: identifying areas for accelerated change*. Ottawa: The Council; 2005.

Once thought of as more of an art than a science, Collaborator competencies are being articulated and translated into learning activities. Assessment tools are evolving to address how physicians seek collaborative opportunities when required, how they determine with whom they should collaborate, and how they demonstrate competence in interprofessional communication and teamwork.

The tools listed below reflect ways to measure the knowledge, skills and attitudes that have been tested in the interprofessional education literature. Limited methodologies have been used to measure competencies to date; the effectiveness of many of the tools is yet to be determined, as rigorous evaluations have not been conducted.

Preferred tools

1. Written tests (short-answer questions, essays)
Of the types of assessment tools that have been studied, the most frequently used are self-assessment questionnaires. This type of written test, conducted before and after an educational intervention, has been used to measure areas including:

1. changes in attitudes or perceptions toward another profession or toward interprofessional collaboration
2. changes in knowledge or skills related to collaboration.

A number of validated questionnaires have been developed. However, it is unclear whether they provide evidence of behavioural change that can be sustainable over time.

2. In-training evaluation reports (ITERs)
Direct observation by physician preceptors using ITERs has typically been used to assess teamwork skills. Although this is a critical aspect of assessment in the clinical setting, "teamwork" has rarely been broken down into its specific components (e.g., knowledge of the roles of other health professionals, effective communication skills). Carefully designed scales that detail the behaviours and skills that inform teamwork would improve the psychometric properties of direct observation.

3. Objective structured clinical examinations (OSCEs)
Scenarios to test learners' abilities to interact and collaborate effectively with other health care practitioners in resolving a conflict or patient care issue can be implemented. Using actors to portray standardized scenarios, a team of learners, including physicians and learners from different health professions, can be put to the test to measure their ability to collaborate in patient-centred team-based OSCE (TOSCE). This type of assessment has been used in a number of settings to measure the acquisition of knowledge and skills related to Collaborator competencies. A standardized checklist or global-rating scale can be used to assess communication skills, clinical decision-making as a team, and role comprehension.

4. Simulation
High-fidelity computerized mannequin simulators have been used to provide objective structured assessments, particularly in acute care settings such as emergency medicine and intensive care. Although expensive, simulation offers the potential to assess collaborative interprofessional work in rare or emergency situations.

5. Multi-source feedback
Multi-source feedback is an attractive option for the assessment of Collaborator activities, as it combines the assessments of multiple team member. However, as with all multi-source assessment, the perspectives and contexts of various contributors need to be carefully considered in forming a global assessment.

Key literature

The assessment literature available for the Collaborator Role is not extensive. Many of the articles available provide evaluation of a program or educational intervention rather than assessment of individual competence. Another inherent weakness within the available literature is that much of the assessment lacks objectiveness in that it is done from a self assessment perspective. However, at this stage, there have been contributions made to the literature to date, which can inform further development of the assessment of the Collaborator Role.

1. Parsell G, Bligh J. The development of a questionnaire to assess the readiness of health care students for interprofessional learning (RIPLS). *Med Educ* 1999;33(2):95-100.

Tool type
Written – SAQ

Study design
Descriptive – tool development

Study population
Undergraduate students (2nd year), 8 health care professions

Comments
This is a description of how a tool (questionnaire) was developed. The description of the process is very useful for other tool development. Utilization of this tool to assess readiness for shared learning should be transferable to multiple contexts (not necessarily large team settings). Although this tool will allow measurement of the effects of the formal educational interventions on learner attitudes, it could also be used with individual learners/practitioners, to assess attitude and to inform dialogue and feedback.

2. Cooper H, Spencer-Dawe E, McLean E. Beginning the process of teamwork: design, implementation and evaluation of an inter-professional education intervention for first year undergraduate students. *J Interprof Care* 2005;19(5):492-508.

Tool type
Written tests: SAQ as part of a program evaluation

Study design
Multi-method study design for evaluation of a learning model

Study population
Undergraduate students – 1st year MD, PT, OT, nursing in an interprofessional learning context

Comments
This article describes an interprofessional learning program intervention with respect to implementation and evaluation. Using Campbell's (2000) phased approach to evaluating complex interventions, the process is described. The description is well done. However, it acknowledges that the structure and logistical organization is necessary for such a program (i.e., multiple disciplines of learners actively interacting together synchronously). Unless this learning context is feasible, the reproducibility of such a program would be difficult. One of the several evaluation tools utilized was the RIPLS (Parcell and Bligh).

3. Singh R, Naughton B, Taylor JS, Koenigsberg MR, Anderson DR, McCausland LL, Wahler RG, et al. A comprehensive collaborative patient safety residency curriculum to address the ACGME core competencies. *Med Educ* 2005;39(12):1195-204.

Tool type
OSCE with multiple stations specific to patient safety content

Study design
single arm descriptive cohort

Study population
Family medicine residents

Comments
This is a description of a curriculum intervention in the area of patient safety with multiple assessment methods. The authors indicate that the results of the OSCE assessment intervention will be reported later. Interestingly, the OSCE is not a single station but multiple stations addressing the competencies (using standardized patients, simulated video analysis, chart review and written stations. However, even without specific evaluation results, several aspects are

discussed and presented that are valuable for the development of direct observation modalities of assessment in the area of collaborator competence. Table 2 is a competency-based assessment blueprint that highlights the ongoing nature of the evaluation in addition to the multiple methods used (including portfolios). The authors also describe a quality assurance component to the curriculum, in which they feel faculty–staff participation is important. They acknowledge the lack of interprofessional involvement among the participants but point out that the planning committee was interprofessional and that the logistical coordination has hampered such involvement to date.

4. Cullen L, Fraser D, Symonds I. Strategies for interprofessional education: the Interprofessional Team Objective Structured Clinical Examination for midwifery and medical students. *Nurse Educ Today* 2003;23(6):427-33.

Tool type

Direct observation: ITOSCE (interprofessional team OSCE)

Study design

Descriptive curriculum design report

Study population

Undergraduate students: medical and midwifery

Comments

This is a description of implementation situated within the area of action research. Although these researchers use a team OSCE as an assessment method, which may be feasible in some contexts, they acknowledge that the process is resource intensive. In addition, in this instance the ITOSCE is being used as a learning model or teaching strategy rather than as an actual assessment tool. Unfortunately, the performance during the ITOSCE (based, however, on a checklist) is not scored, but is used only as a means to stimulate formative feedback by the facilitator. Evaluations of interprofessional learning are self-reported perceptions. This strategy and even the concept of the team OSCE is likely most useful if an interprofessional team learning or practice context exists.

5. Ritchie PD, Cameron PA. An evaluation of trauma team leader performance by video recording. *Aust NZ J Surg* 1999;69(3):183-6.

Tool type

Direct observation with videotape assessment

Study design

Cross-sectional cohort

Study population
Emergency physicians and emergency and surgical residents (Australia)

Comments
This publication illuminates the fact that using video for later analysis (evaluation and feedback) is possible in less traditional settings (in the emergency department as compared to a family medicine residency program environment, where utilization is quite high). The authors point out considerations specifically related to videotaping, such as patient confidentiality, patient and participant consent and medicolegal implications, as well as logistical issues related to taping. There is also some discussion about the initial hesitancy among participants that did not ultimately interfere with implementation. In fact, they report general acceptance of the tool in the end.

---

6. Fichtner CG, Hardy D, Patel M, Stout CE, Simpatico TA, Dove H, Cook LP, Grossman LS, Giffort DW. A self-assessment program for multidisciplinary mental health teams. *Psychiatr Serv* 2001;52(10):1352-7.

Tool type
Multi-source feedback

Study design
Cohort, cross-sectional

Study population
Health care professions, in mental health, 7 disciplines

Comments
Although this publication is specific to the mental health care context, the more limiting factor may be the context of team-based delivery of care. The SLATE tool, however, has more generalized potential for assessment of collaboration competency in team contexts. The tool emphasizes the physician as the team leader, but with a recognition that this needs to be a collaborative leadership. Sixteen (16) of the 42 items on the scale are directed toward the team leadership and the behaviours associated with facilitating collaboration. In this study, the tool was not specifically used for program evaluation tool but rather to stimulate team reflection. The authors acknowledge that the psychometric properties (including reliability and validity) of the scale's internal structure have not yet been established.

Other literature

Anderson E, Manek N, Davidson A. Evaluation of a model for maximizing interprofessional education in an acute hospital. *J Interprof Care* 2006:20(2):182-94.

Bateman B, Wilson FC, Bingham D. Team effectiveness – development of an audit questionnaire. *J Manage Dev* 2002:21(3/4),215-6.

Carpenter J, Barnes D, Dickinson C, Wooff D. Outcomes of interprofessional education for community mental health services in England: the longitudinal evaluation of a postgraduate programme. *J Interprof Care* 2006:20(2):145-61.

DeVita MA, Schaefer J, Lutz J, Wang H, Dongilli T. Improving medical emergency team (MET) performance using a novel curriculum and a computerized human patient simulator. *Qual Saf Health Care* 2005:14(5):326-31.

Fallsberg MB, Wijma K. Student attitudes towards the goals of an interprofessional training ward. *Med Teach* 1999:21(6):576-81.

Farrell M, Ryan S, Langrick B. Breaking bad news within a paediatric setting: an evaluation report of a collaborative education workshop to support health professionals *J Adv Nurs* 2001:36(6):765-75.

Fichtner CG, Stout CE, Dove H, Lardon CS. Psychiatric leadership and the clinical team: simulated in vivo treatment planning performance as teamwork proxy and learning laboratory. *Adm Policy Ment Health* 2000:27(5):313-37.

Fineberg IC. Preparing professionals for family conferences in palliative care: evaluation results of an interdisciplinary approach. *J Palliat Med* 2005:8(4):857-66.

Fineberg IC, Wenger NS, Forrow L. Interdisciplinary education: evaluation of a palliative care training intervention for pre-professionals. *Acad Med* 2004;79(8):769-76.

Harward DH, Tresolini CP, Davis WA. Can participation in a health affairs interdisciplinary case conference improve medical students' knowledge and attitudes? *Acad Med* 2006:81(3):257-61.

Hyer K, Fairchild S, Abraham I, Mezey M, Fulmer T. Measuring attitudes related to interdisciplinary training: revising the Heinemann, Schmitt & Farell attitudes toward health care teams scale. *JIC* 2000:14(3): 249-58

Johnson D and Cujec B Comparison of self, nurse, andphysician assessment of residents rotating through an intensive careunit.[see comment]. *Crit Care Med* 1998:26(11):1811-6.

Luecht RM, Madsen MK, Taugher MP, Petterson BJ. Assessing professional perceptions: design and validation of an interdisciplinary education perception scale. *J Allied Health*,1990:19,181-91

Potter TB and Palmer RG. 360-degree assessment in a multidisciplinary team setting. *Rheumatology* 2003:42 (11):1404-7.

Reeves S, Freeth D The London training ward: an innovative interprofessional learning initiative. *J Interprof Care*, 2002:16(1)41-52.

Schreiber MA, Holcomb JB, Conaway CW, Campbell KD, Wall M, Mattox KL. Military trauma training performed in a civilian trauma center. *J Surg Res*, 2002:104(1),8-14

Small SD, Wuerz RC, Simon R, Shapiro N, Conn A, Setnik G. Demonstration of high-fidelity simulation team training for emergency medicine. *Acad.Emerg.Med.* 1999;6(4):312-23.

Ummenhofer W et al. Team Performance in the emergency room: assessment of inter-disciplinary attitudes. *Resuscitation* 2001;49(1):39-46.

3.5 Manager

Saleem Razack and Deepak Dath

Definition

As Managers, physicians are integral participants in health care organizations, organizing sustainable practices, making decisions about allocating resources and contributing to the effectiveness of the health care system.

Key competencies

Physicians are able to ...

1. Participate in activities that contribute to the effectiveness of their health care organizations and systems;
2. Manage their practice and career effectively;
3. Allocate finite health care resources appropriately;
4. Serve in administration and leadership roles, as appropriate.

Overview

In modern health care, physicians often hold multifaceted clinical, administrative, research and educational leadership positions. As professionals, they are expected to contribute to the welfare of their communities. Physicians must also achieve balance between these multiple activities and their personal and family commitments. To succeed in these simultaneous responsibilities, physicians must acquire and maintain good managerial skills. They must manage their practices and develop their careers, show leadership, allocate resources and participate in the organizational dynamics of the health care system.

Although the body of literature supporting the physician Manager Role is nascent, the articles annotated below are highlighted as examples that will help the reader to get started.

Most learners begin their medical education with no previous management training. Therefore, the management skills they have at the beginning of their careers will have been acquired during medical training. Postgraduate programs have a mandate to ensure that learners are well prepared for the specific managerial responsibilities that their graduates will be expected to fulfill. Regular assessment of the Manager Role is necessary for programs to understand what trainees learn, how well they have learned it, and how these programs can improve Manager education. The methods a program employs to teach management skills will influence the method of assessment. Although several types of assessment lend themselves to the task of evaluating residents as

Managers; none stand alone as a standard or as a complete method of assessment. All require significant work, and some have significant drawbacks. How some of these can apply to the Manager Role is outlined below.

Preferred tools

1. Multi-source feedback and peer evaluation
The use of "360-degree evaluation" has been adopted by some business corporations to evaluate and provide feedback on management skills. Adopted by medical educators and renamed multi-source feedback, it lends itself well to the assessment of all the key competencies of the Manager Role. Assessors who are junior or senior to a learner can evaluate how that learner behaves in the hierarchy and whether the learner is functioning appropriately, prioritizing and delegating tasks, exhibiting leadership qualities, planning for the future, making the best use of time and resources, etc. Allied health professionals, patients and others can assess the learner's interaction, communication and leadership to round out the assessment. Physicians from other consultative services may be able to assess how the learner uses and allocates resources in the system.

Multi-source feedback design needs to include specific questions that address each of the key competencies of the Manager Role. This assessment method can be computerized to improve efficiency and feasibility.

2. Simulation
Simulation can be used to assess a learner's ability to handle complex, critical situations. Simulation scenarios can be simple or complex and can involve single learners or teams. Complex simulations involving multiple learners and high-fidelity computer-driven mannequins require the learner to provide leadership, delegate tasks, communicate, provide feedback, plan, make difficult decisions, etc. All of these skills are incorporated into the Manager Role.

This tool is particularly useful for assessing management competence relating to patient care.

3. Portfolio
The management literature emphasizes a reflective approach to learning and assessment. To support this approach, assessment portfolios can include items such as committee work, practice organization innovations, audits and quality assurance projects, along with reflections generated by these experiences. The strength of portfolios is that they aid both the assessment of how management principles are applied to real situations and the reflection that promotes longitudinal learning.

Practice and career management can also be assessed through the inclusion of curricula vitae and narrative reviews of discussions with academic mentors.

4. Direct observation
Learners can demonstrate managerial skills in many clinical scenarios. They must be able to balance competing demands, whether professional or personal.
Time management can be demonstrated through timely attendance at mandatory activities, efficient patient management, infrequent changes or oversight shifts in scheduling, and adequate rest for optimal functioning. Supervisors can observe effective mobilization of health care resources and appropriate delegation to other team members during clinics, inpatient ward activities and emergency department shifts. Surgical learners can be assessed on their ability to properly manage the booking and movement of patients through the operating theatre on busy case days.

Key literature

1. Rodgers KG, Manifold C. 360-degree feedback: possibilities for assessment of the ACGME core competencies for emergency medicine residents. *Acad Emerg Med* 2002;9(11):1300-4.

Tool type
Multi-source feedback

Study design
Description of a new instrument

Study population
No participants

Comments
This article is a thought piece that helps bridge the gap between an approach designed for businesses and its application to graduate medical education. A review of the background will give a program director a good flavour of the intricacies involved in implementing this tool in a residency program. It does not specifically address management competencies and, in fact, states that this tool may not be the best choice for rating the key competencies of the Manager Role in the CanMEDS 2005 Framework. Many sources of further information are cited. Thoughtful conclusions are stated.

---

2. Higgins RS, Bridges J, Burke JM, O'Donnell MA, Cohen NM, Wilkes SB. Implementing the ACGME general competencies in a cardiothoracic surgery residency program using 360-degree feedback. *Ann Thorac Surg* 2004;77(1):12-7.

Tool type
Multi-source feedback

Study design
Prospective, program description

Study population
Senior cardiothoracic surgery residents

Comments

This article is useful in a number of ways. It shows that 360-degree evaluations are possible in residency programs, outlines how one program implemented the process, describes clearly the development of the instrument and discusses some pitfalls. There are management components in the evaluation instrument, although the instrument was meant to assess the entire ACGME competency spectrum. The authors stated how they applied the instrument, how they used the results and how they expected the exercise to benefit the residents. Clearly, this is a description, not a recipe, and does not provide evidence of benefit. However, at this stage of competency assessment it provides useful guidance for residency programs interested in implementing these types of evaluations.

3. O'Sullivan PS, Reckase MD, McClain T, Savidge MA, Clardy JA et al. Demonstration of portfolios to assess competency of residents. *Adv Health Scie Ed* 2005;9(4):309-23.

Tool type

Portfolios

Study design

Cross-sectional Study

Study population

PGY 1–4 residents

Comments

Portfolio assessment is another tool that is difficult to use properly in a residency program. These authors demonstrate that diligent planning can result in a successful implementation of a portfolio assessment. Much of the planning is detailed in the article, and the authors describe problems and pitfalls that had to be overcome. The definitions and guidelines they used to determine what residents could include in the portfolio are not included in the study. The guidelines for raters are also absent. The study showed that the psychometric properties of using the portfolio for assessment were good at the decision-making level. This study did not specifically address management issues, but the description of the implementation of this assessment suggests that management issues could be defined and included at the discretion of the program director.

4. Collins J, Amsel S, Alderson PO. Teaching noninterpretive skills to radiology residents: a collaborative effort between the American College of Radiology and the Association of Program Directors in Radiology. *Acad Radiol* 2001;8:903–7.

Tool type

Written examination

Study design
Prospective intervention, pre–post design

Study population
Radiology residents

Comments
Although this study focuses more on an education intervention, it does include a pre–post written test design to assess learning. It also describes some non-clinical factors important for resident education, such as financial aspects of practice management and accreditation processes.

Other literature

Arnold L. Assessing professional behaviors: Yesterday, today, and tomorrow. *Acad Med* 2002;77:502-15

Byrne AJ, Sellen AJ, Jones JG. Errors on anesthetic record charts as measure of performance during simulated critical incidents. *Br J Anesth* 1998;80:58-62.

Challis M. AMEE medical education guide no. 11 (revised): Portfolio-based learning and assessment in medical education. *Med Teach* 1999;21:370-86.

Hall W, Violato C, Lewkonia R et al. Assessment of physician performance in Alberta: The physician achievement review. *CMAJ* 1999;161:52-7.

Norcini JJ. The mini clinical evaluation exercise (mini-CEX). *Clin Teach* 2005;2:25-9.

Norcini JJ, Blank LL, Duffy D, Fortna GS. The Mini-CEX: a method for assessing clinical skills. *Ann Intern Med* 2003;138:476-81.

Murray WB, Foster PA. Crisis resource management among strangers: principles of organizing a multidiciplinary group for crisis resource management. *J Clinical Anesth* 2000;12:633-8.

Norman G. *Evaluation methods: a resource handbook*. Hamilton (ON): Program for Educational Development, McMaster University; 1995. p. 71-7.

Potter TB, Palmer RG. 360-degree assessment in a multidisciplinary team setting. *Rheumatology* 2003;42(11):1404-7.

Useful website

www.ccl.org
Center for Creative Leadership, Greensboro(NC)

3.6 Health Advocate

Sarita Verma and Glen Bandiera

Definition

As Health Advocates, physicians responsibly use their expertise and influence to advance the health and well-being of individual patients, communities and populations.

Key competencies

Physicians are able to ...

1. Respond to individual patient health needs and issues as part of patient care;
2. Respond to the health needs of the communities that they serve;
3. Identify the determinants of health of the populations that they serve;
4. Promote the health of individual patients, communities and populations.

Overview

Effective, comprehensive patient care requires the recognition and appreciation of determinants of health. The Health Advocacy Role allows for a spectrum of responses to issues related to health determinants—at the individual level, in the community and at a societal level. Physicians as health advocates must be responsible in their use of authority and influence and in mobilizing needed resources. This Role requires active participation in the health care system and is foundational in the balancing of competing Roles. In 2005, the Health Advocate Role was revised to focus on "physician influence and health care system knowledge for patient care."

In clinical training, the varied faces of advocacy appear in different rotations and circumstances. The teaching and assessment of advocacy must fit with standard professional practices in these areas. Patients need physicians to assist them in navigating through the health care system and accessing appropriate health resources in a timely manner. Advocating for investigations, advising on appropriate changes to a care plan, mobilizing community resources and discussing risk-factor modification are examples. Communities and societies need physicians' special expertise to identify and collaboratively address broad health issues and the determinants of health. Specialty-specific activities may involve prevention initiatives, policy or guideline development and lobbying for change at the community level.

Preferred tools

1. Essays

Advocacy initiatives can be hard for supervisors to identify: they often occur between learner and patient, or between the learner and other health care professionals, and may also occur outside the clinical rotation. Essays allow learners to report on their own experiences, to increase their awareness of the Role, and to engage in self-reflection. Learners are expected to answer a question and discuss the issues clearly and logically, having researched the topic or reflected on personal experience. Having learners describe how they acted as health advocates in their own practice and observed health advocacy in action through the example of other physicians can provide insight into their understanding of the Role. Essays can be marked as a test or incorporated into a portfolio.

2. Short-answer questions (SAQs)
Knowledge components of the Health Advocate Role are easily tested in this format. SAQs have the distinct advantage of assessing the unassisted recall (rather than recognition) of information. Questions relating to risk factors for disease, options for injury and disease prevention, and pro-and-con arguments for proposed or enacted legislation are particularly well suited to the SAQ format. SAQs can be incorporated into rotations or in-training examinations, or can form the basis for a specific Health Advocate examination after a workshop or project.

3. Direct observation and In-Training Evaluation Reports (ITERs)
Items related to the appreciation of determinants of health and to patient advocacy can be included on ITERs. Assessors can be asked how often learners identify and address risk factors and how effectively they advocate for patients within the system. However, it is inappropriate to use ITERs for advocacy initiatives that would not be expected to arise during routine activities on a given rotation. For example, although learners may be expected to understand the process whereby legislation is passed and how to involve themselves in community and societal debate, this sphere of activity might not be possible at an ambulatory clinic.

A learner's ability to go the extra step in clinical care, such as seeking out drug coverage for a patient unable to afford the medication of best evidence, engaging allied health professionals in the betterment of service for patients, or advocating for home care, placement, or later discharge from hospital are all measures of performance in the Health Advocate Role.

4. Objective structured clinical evaluations (OSCEs) and standardized patients
Simulation testing allows a specific skill set to be explicitly assessed in isolation from other competing demands and provides an opportunity for directed feedback. Learners can be presented with health advocacy challenges during OSCE stations. The skills involved in eliciting relevant risk factors, discussing risk modification, educating patients, and obtaining access to clinical resources can be assessed in this format. Standardized patients can be very effective in prompting learners to identify advocacy issues and in revealing the resourcefulness and problem-solving ability to advocate for patients with multifactorial problems, both acute and chronic. Assessment can be done in a global fashion or with checklists of specific behaviours and may or may not involve the standardized patients as assessors.

5. Multi-source feedback and peer evaluations

Although little has been written about the use of multi-source feedback to assess the Health Advocate Role, this method of assessment has many theoretical advantages. Numerous sources of information could form the basis for such an assessment: patients, families, nurses, consultants, peers and allied health professionals can be recruited to provide input on the learner's specific advocacy activities. Behaviour related to discharge planning, multidisciplinary rounds, family meetings, consultation requests, clinical care discussions and presentations on health promotion and disease prevention might be included in such assessments.

6. Portfolios

Portfolios allow a chronology of learner advocacy activities to develop over the course of several years. Portfolios might include letters, newspaper articles on advocacy, or evidence of involvement with special interest groups, political activities and government. Ideally, each component of the portfolio would contain an element of self-reflection. Essays about clinical encounters would also be appropriate. Evidence of advocacy activity relevant to the specialty could be collected and assessed across the training period, using a quantitative, qualitative or combined approach to gauge the frequency, extent, quality and effectiveness of advocacy involvement. The portfolio would be part of an overall assessment at the time of eligibility for certification.

Key literature

1. Bandiera GW. Emergency medicine health advocacy. *Can J Emerg Med* 2003;5(5): 336-42

Tool type

Written exam (essay) and portfolios (variant)

Study design

Single-arm descriptive report

Study population

Emergency medicine residents

Comments

This article describes a three-part curriculum to stimulate interest and activity in health advocacy. Residents discussed multiple examples of advocacy relevant to their specialty, provided a critique of various advocacy examples provided as study material and, finally, wrote a brief essay and critique on their own personal practice experience with advocacy. The latter was presented to their peers for discussion. The evaluation of the essays was not described, but formal processes to accomplish this or inclusion of the essays in an overall residency portfolio could easily be achieved.

2. Borgiel AEM, Williams JL, Davis DA, Dunn EV, Hobbs N, Hutchinson B, et al. Evaluating the effectiveness of 2 educational interventions in family practice. *CMAJ* 1999;161(8): 965-70.

Tool type

Practice-based assessment, chart review, patient survey

Study design

Randomized controlled trial

Study population

Family practitioners

Comments

Although this study was designed to determine the effects of two different educational interventions on the preventive health practices of family physicians, it used some innovative and well-described tools to carry out the evaluation. The investigators asked patients to complete surveys. Completed chart reviews were performed before and after the educational interventions. There was no difference based on the type of intervention, but the investigators did demonstrate that the tools were capable of providing insight into subjects' practices.

3. Brill JR, Ohly S, Stearns MA. Training community-responsive physicians. 2002;*Acad Med* 77(7):747.

Tool type

Portfolios and global assessment forms

Study design

Descriptive curriculum design

Study population

Family practice residents

Comments

This is an innovative study that reports the use of a formal curriculum in health advocacy intended to stimulate interest in rural practice and public health. Residents were expected to produce written summaries for inclusion in a portfolio and undertake periodic assessments of their activities using a predefined series of eight specific content domains.

4. Leone RJ, Hammond JS. Surgical residents' knowledge of injury prevention principles. *Am J Surg* 2000;180(3):223-6.

Tool type
Written test

Study design
Cross-sectional study

Study population
General surgery residents at three sites

Comments
This is one of the few studies that focus on assessment rather than teaching methods. It describes a written short-answer test used to assess surgery residents' knowledge of injury prevention, injury patterns and intentional violence. Residents generally performed poorly, yet demonstrated an interest in learning more about the area.

5. Verma S, Flynn L, Seguin R. Faculty's and residents' perceptions of teaching and evaluating the role of health advocate: a study at one Canadian university. *Acad Med* 2005;80(1):103-8.

Tool type
Practice-based assessment (variant)

Study design
Focus group qualitative study

Study population
Canadian postgraduate medical residents

Comments
Faculty and residents participated in separate focus groups to determine their level of understanding of the Health Advocate Role and its assessment. Although not an assessment paper per se, this study does provide insight into the current level of understanding about the challenges faced by both faculty and residents in addressing the need to teach and assess residents as health advocates. Curriculum developers could turn this focus group design into a self-study or portfolio-based assessment technique by having residents record their experiences and report them to a group or during a one-on-one meeting with their program director or faculty advisor. Interestingly, the authors found that, although faculty saw the Health Advocate Role as integral to their professional lives and as something that should be apparent to learners, residents were unaware of the role health advocacy played in their faculty members' practices.

Other literature

Aitken ME, Rowlands LA, Wheeler JG. Advocating for children's health at the state level. *Arch Pediatr Adolesc Med* 2001;155 (8): 877-80.

Brill JR, Ohly S, Stearns MA. Training community-responsive physicians. *Acad Med* 2002;77(7): 747.

Borgiel AEM, Williams JL, Davis DA, Dunn EV, Hobbs N, Hutchinson B, et al. Evaluating the effectiveness of 2 educational interventions in family practice. *CMAJ* 1999;161(8):965-70.

Clark PA. What residents are not learning: observations in an NICU. *Acad Med* 76 2001;(5): 419-24.

Frank JR, Langer B. Collaboration, communication, management, and advocacy: teaching surgeons new skills through CanMEDS project. *World J Surg* 2003;27:972-8.

Kilduff A, McKeown K, Crowther A (1998) Health needs assessment in primary care: the evolution of practical public health approach. *Public Health* 112(3):175-81.

Leone RJ,Hammond JS. Surgical residents' knowledge of injury prevention principles. *Am J Surg* 2000;180(3):223-6.

Notzer N, Abramovitz R. Clinical learning experiences of Israeli medical students in health promotion and prevention of cancer and cardiovascular diseases. *Isr Med Assoc J* 2002;4(2):149-52.

Oandasan I, Barker KK. Educating for advocacy: exploring the source and substance of community-responsive physicians. *Acad Med* 2003;78(10 Suppl):S16-S19.

Taylor KL, Chudley AE. Meeting the needs of future physicians: a core curriculum initiative for postgraduate medical education at a Canadian university. *Med Educ* 2001;35(10):973-82.

Verma S, Flynn L, Seguin R. Faculty's and residents' perceptions of teaching and evaluating the role of health advocate: a study at one Canadian university. *Acad Med* 2005;80(1):103-8.

Wilson A, McDonald P. Comparison of patient questionnaire, medical record, and audio tape in assessment of health promotion in general practice consultations. *BMJ* 1994;309:1483-5.

3.7 Scholar

Jonathan Sherbino

Definition

As Scholars, physicians demonstrate a lifelong commitment to reflective learning, as well as the creation, dissemination, application and translation of medical knowledge.

Key competencies

Physicians are able to ...

1. Maintain and enhance professional activities through ongoing learning;
2. Critically evaluate information and its sources, and apply this appropriately to practice decisions;
3. Facilitate the learning of patients, families, students, residents, other health professionals, the public, and others, as appropriate;
4. Contribute to the creation, dissemination, application, and translation of new medical knowledge and practices.

Overview

The CanMEDS Scholar Role encompasses diverse competencies, including lifelong learning, critical appraisal (e.g., evidence-based practice), teaching and research. These elements support a competent clinical practice (lifelong learning and critical appraisal) and contribute to the advancement of the profession (research and teaching).

Despite the significance of the Scholar Role, little research has been directed toward the teaching and assessment of its component competencies. Curriculum development and curriculum evaluation related to continuing professional development is widely available in the literature, yet the assessment of behaviours related to lifelong learning are not extensively studied. There is also a dearth of literature on assessment tools to gauge competence in the researcher role, despite the fact that the assessment of research skills is intrinsic to any study and is reflected in grant application reviews and manuscript peer reviews. Finally, there are several excellent systematic reviews outlining components of successful teaching in medicine. However, research supporting associated assessment tools specific to medical teaching is uncommon. Sophisticated teaching assessments have been described in the higher-education literature, but clinical teachers and educators require translation of these tools before they can be applied in the medical education environment. In contrast to the limited publication of assessment tools for lifelong learning and research competencies, critical appraisal assessment tools are easily found in the literature.

Recognizing these challenges, some tools seem preferentially suited to assessment of the Scholar Role. As with all CanMEDS Roles, no single tool is sufficient to assess all of the key Scholar competencies. Therefore, multiple assessors using multiple tools should be used to ensure a valid and reliable assessment of learners. The following four tools are felt to be most appropriate in the assessment of the Scholar Role.

Preferred tools

1. Portfolios
Portfolios are well suited to assess the Scholar Role. They are by definition a longitudinal tool, which matches them well with the lifelong learner competency. Self-learning projects with associated reflective pieces can readily be used to assess the progress of a trainee. Brief synopses of seminars, lectures or clinical teaching encounters (performed by the learner) with associated teaching scores would be excellent additions to a portfolio. Finally, a representative sample (e.g., literature review, grant application, manuscript with related peer reviews) of a research project would also serve the assessment of research competency.

2. Short-answer questions (SAQs)
SAQs are an effective and efficient means to assess several of the competencies that constitute the Scholar Role. Learners could be required to critically appraise a specialty-specific study and to answer associated questions. Other uses might include requesting the appropriate research methodology and study design for a given research question, asking for a list of criteria for quality study design or requesting simple calculations of basic statistical results.

3. Direct observation and in-training evaluation reports (ITERs)
Direct observation of a learner's critical appraisal (e.g., article presentation at journal club) or teaching skills is easily accomplished. Real behaviour, in real time, is assessed. Research supervisors could similarly assess learners through direct observation. However, if only a small number of research supervisors are incorporated into the assessment, the reliability of direct observation is restricted. Direct observation is a poor choice for assessing the lifelong learning competency. The related observable behaviours and longitudinal nature of this competency do not match the strengths of this assessment tool. The use of global assessment scales or checklist scores should be determined by the particular behaviours assessed.

4. Multi-source feedback and peer assessment
Multi-source feedback has some utility in assessing the Scholar Role. In particular, this tool is able to assess teaching competency. The challenge with this tool is in designing a questionnaire that appropriately captures teaching behaviour. Peers, allied health professionals and patients might not readily identify as "teaching" the facilitation of learning that routinely occurs during clinical encounters. Distinguishing these "teaching moments" (e.g., explaining the pathophysiology of an illness to a patient, discussing the therapeutic benefits of one medication

versus another with a nursing colleague) from traditional lectures or seminars is vital in capturing valid assessments from multiple sources. The inclusion of peer evaluation is common for traditional teaching venues (e.g., rounds) and for clinical (i.e., bedside) teaching between senior and junior learners. The inclusion of true peer assessment (involving learners at identical stages of training) for teaching behaviours surrounding a clinical case poses unique challenges. Case discussions might not be identified as teaching moments, and the assessment may lack validity.

Key literature

1. Stern DT, Linzer M, O'Sullivan PS, Weld L. Evaluating medical residents' literature-appraisal skills. *Acad Med* 1995; 70(2):152-4.

Tool type
Self-report, direct observation

Study design
Prospective interventional, single cohort

Study population
Medical residents

Comments
Despite methodological flaws and equivocal findings, this study provides a good example of a written exam tool used to assess critical appraisal skills. A component of self-reflection is also included, demonstrating how these data could be incorporated into a portfolio.

2. Fliegel JE, Frohna JG, Mangrulkar RS. A computer-based OSCE station to measure competence in evidence-based medicine skills in medical students. *Acad Med* 2002;77(11):1157-8.

Tool type
Simulated case / objective structured clinical evaluation (OSCE), written examination

Study design
Prospective intervention, single cohort

Study population
Medical students

Comments
This study uses a written exam to assess critical appraisal skills and measures the psychometric properties of the tool specific to this assessment environment. Of interest, this paper demonstrates how such an assessment tool could be incorporated into an OSCE.

3. Snell L, Tallet S, Haist S, Hays R, Norcini J, Prince K, et al. A review of the evaluation of clinical teaching: new perspectives and challenges. *Med Educ* 2000; 34(10):862-70.

Tool type
Multiple-source feedback (MSF)

Study design
Review article

Study population
Medical teachers

Comments
This narrative review provides a solid theoretical ground for assessment of the teaching competency. Of interest, the review indirectly suggests the utility of MSF as an assessment tool for teaching skills.

4. Katz NT, McCarty-Gillespie L, Magrane DM. Direct observation as a tool for needs assessment of resident teaching skills in the ambulatory setting. *Am J Obstet Gynecol* 2004;189(3):684-7.

Tool type
Direct observation (checklist)

Study design
Interventional, single cohort

Study population
Medical residents

Comments
This study evaluated a direct observation teaching assessment tool that used a checklist scoring system. The study findings demonstrated that teaching behaviours did not improve with level of training. The authors concluded that this lack of improvement reflected curriculum deficiencies. However, the findings might also be a function of the insensitivity of the checklist scoring system—a consideration for the design of other direct observation teaching assessment tools.

5. Jackson JL, O'Malley PG, Salerno SM. The Teacher and Learner Interactive Assessment System (TeLIAS): a new tool to assess teaching behaviours in the ambulatory setting. *Teach Learn Med* 2002;14(4):249-56.

Tool type
Direct observation (audiotaped)

Study design
Observational, qualitative

Study population
Medical students

Comments
The assessment tool described in this study, which concerns clinical (bedside) teaching, is not immediately applicable to learner assessment. However, its finding could inform the development of a specialty-specific direct observation tool.

Other literature

Braxtton JM, Del Favero M. Evaluating scholarship performance: traditional and emergent assessment templates. *N Dir Teach Learn* 2002; (114):19-31.

Carusetta E. Evaluating teaching through teaching awards. *N Dir Teach Learn* 2001; (88):31-40.

Cramer JS, Mahoney MC. Introducing evidence based medicine to the journal club, using a structured pre and post test: a cohort study. *BMC Med Educ* 2001; 1(6) [Epub Nov 6]

Hojat M, Nasca TJ, Erdmann JB, Fribsy AJ, Veloski JJ, Connella JS. An operational measure of physician lifelong learning: its development, components and preliminary psychometric data. *Med Teach* 2003; 25(4)433-7.

Ramos KD, Schafer S, Tracz SM. Validation of the Fresno test of competence in evidence based medicine. *BMJ* 2003; 326:319-21.

Shelvin M et al. The validity of student evaluation of teaching in higher education: love me, love my lectures? *Assess Eval Higher Educ* 2000; 25(4):397-405.

Wiese J, Varosy P, Tierney L. Improving oral presentation skills with a clinical reasoning curriculum: a prospective controlled study. *Am J Med* 2002; 112(3):212-8.

3.8 Professional

Ramona A. Kearney, Derek Puddester and Jason R. Frank

Definition

As Professionals, physicians are committed to the health and well-being of individuals and society through ethical practice, profession-led regulation and high personal standards of behaviour.

Key competencies

Physicians are able to ...

1. Demonstrate a commitment to their patients, profession, and society through ethical practice;
2. Demonstrate a commitment to their patients, profession, and society through participation in profession-led regulation;
3. Demonstrate a commitment to physician health and sustainable practice.

Overview

As members of an independent profession accorded the privileges of clinical autonomy and self-regulation, today's physicians are trusted to place concern for the welfare of their patients and society as a whole above their own interests. It is only through the continued demonstration of commitment to ethical practice and the maintenance of regulatory standards that this fiduciary relationship with society will be sustained and physicians will continue to be viewed by society as valued, competent and autonomous professionals.

Professionalism refers to both the behaviours of individuals and the core values that the profession has internalized. Competence in the Professional Role has been learned mainly through the informal and hidden curricula of medical schools. Professionalism is often thought to develop in physicians simply by completing the training process, at the end of which one is deemed to have "become" a professional. This fails to recognize that the training environment can be hostile and can induce cynicism and decayed moral reasoning. Recently, professionalism has come under scrutiny by society, and threats to professionalism have been identified. Educators have recognized that an explicit curriculum of competencies in this domain and associated assessment paradigms are needed.

The CanMEDS Professional Role is uniquely organized around three key competencies. The first deals with the behaviours of ethical practice—the domain most educators think of when they consider "professionalism." There is a large body of literature on approaches to assessing this domain. Assessments can take place in the clinical environment, where observations by many colleagues and co-workers can provide a full picture of the individual's professionalism. Since reflection is fundamental to learning, and professionalism is a developmental process, assessments that look at trainees' reflections may be a valuable source of information on their emerging professionalism.

The second key competency deals with the abilities of physicians to practise effectively within the bounds of a self-regulating profession. There is little in the literature that describes approaches to assessing this. However, these behaviours are well-suited to assessment through portfolios, and the underlying knowledge base can be assessed using written tests.

Finally, the third key competency of the CanMEDS Professional Role addresses the necessary abilities to have an effective, sustainable practice. Members of the profession have been concerned about physician health and well-being for well over a century. In recent decades, the profession has overtly acknowledged the need for formal training in personal health and well-being, resiliency, sustainability, and personal and career development. Again, portfolios are well suited to track development in this domain, and written tests can be employed to capture the underlying relevant knowledge base.

Preferred tools

The tools that best assess professionalism are those that look at behaviour in the workplace and those that assess the development of professionalism in the individual through reflection. The preferred tools for the assessment of behaviour are:

1. Direct observation and in-training evaluation reports (ITERs)
Direct observation of actual practice provides the highest fidelity in assessing aspects of professionalism. Assessment of behaviour can occur throughout the learner's training and provide insight into the development of professionalism, especially if a small group of assessors is involved in assessing many in-training situations. Forms can be designed with lists of explicit behaviours listed and scales representing either frequency ("never" to "always") and quality ("poor" to "excellent") or the extent to which expectations are met. Specific items might relate to handling ethical issues (such as patient autonomy and confidentiality), self-awareness, responsibility and fulfilling a duty to care.

2. Multi-source feedback
Multi-source feedback allows input from a variety of colleagues and co-workers to provide many snapshots of behaviour under different circumstances. The breadth of behaviour can be assessed through this method, as opposed to the depth often assessed through In-Training Evaluation Reports (ITERs). Validity is attained through a large number of assessments, and the careful selection of contributors will add to face validity. Patients and families can attest to frank discussions and autonomy, nurses can comment on delegation of medical acts and respectful interprofessional relationships, and direct supervisors can assess receptiveness to feedback and self-assessment. Peers might be a good source of feedback on learner well-being and the behaviours of sustainable practice.

3. Portfolios
Portfolios allow insight into the core of the developing professional by tracking growth through reflection. They provide feedback for the learner, who can set his or her own goals for development and assess progress. Portfolios are also useful for identifying deficiencies and are therefore useful in remediation. Inclusions might take the form of short essays on the resolution of ethical issues, personal experiences with duties to care, letters attesting to involvement in regulatory or policy-making bodies, or self-determined goals for personal development with follow-up assessments of success.

Key literature

1. Arnold L. Assessing professional behaviour: yesterday, today, and tomorrow. *Acad Med* 2002; 77(6):502-15.

Tool type
Various

Study design
Systematic review

Study population
Mixed (undergraduate, postgraduate, non-medical)

Comments
This is an excellent review of the assessment of professionalism. The author describes measurement tools from studies on assessment of professional behaviour as part of clinical performance, on professional behaviour alone and on separate elements of humanisms and self-reflection. It provides numerous assessment tools with a discussion of the associated psychometric properties of each tool.

2. Larkin GL, Binder L, Houry D, Adams J. Defining and evaluating professionalism: a core competency for graduate emergency medicine education. *Acad Emerg Med* 2002; 9(11):1249-56.

Tool design
Various

Study design
Consensus statement

Study population
Postgraduate, emergency medicine

Comments

This article provides a consensus list of professional behaviours. It also structures assessment tools of professionalism according to a hierarchy spanning knowledge to behaviour: "knows," "knows how" and "shows how."

---

3. Lynch DC, Surdyk PM, Eiser AR. Assessing professionalism: a review of the literature. *Med Teach* 2004; 26(4):366-73.

Tool design

Various

Study design

Systematic review

Study population

Mixed (undergraduate, postgraduate)

Comments

This comprehensive review has a particular focus on medical ethics. It also provides general recommendations for assessing professionalism and specific recommendations for assessing residents and practising physicians.

---

4. Ginsburg S, Regehr G, Hatala R, McNaughton N, Frohna A, Hodges B, et al. Context, conflict, and resolution: a new conceptual framework for evaluating professionalism. *Acad Med* 2000; 75(10):S6-S11.

Tool design

Various

Study design

Systematic review

Study population

Mixed (undergraduate, postgraduate)

Comments

This paper reviews the literature on the types of evaluative instruments used for measuring professionalism in medical education and outlines fundamental conceptual deficiencies that exist in this literature. They argue that the three most important missing components are consideration of the contexts in which unprofessional behaviours occur, the conflicts that lead to these lapses, and the reasons students make the choices they make. They then propose strategies for resolving these issues.

Other literature

The CMA Centre on Physician Health and Well Being, a virtual centre housed at www.cma.ca, has identified a large number of resources, documents and studies that can be readily accessed from their website. The following references may be of particular value for postgraduate training:

Books

Goldman LS, Myers M, Dickstein LJ, editors. T*he handbook of physician health: the essential guide to understanding the health care needs of physicians.* Chicago: American Medical Association; 2000

Peterkin A. *Staying human during residency training.* 3rd ed. Toronto: University of Toronto, 2004.

Stern DT. *Measuring medical professionalism*; 2006. New York: Oxford University Press; 2006.

Journals, booklets, policy statements

Puddester D, editor. Creating a healthy culture in medicine: Report of the 2004 AMA/CMA International Conference on Physician Health. Ottawa: Canadian Medical Association, 2005 Available: www.cma.ca

Canadian Medical Association. Physician health and well-being [policy statement]. Available: http://www.cma.ca/index.cfm/ci_id/3211/la_id/1.htm

Western Journal of Medicine 2001;174(1). Special issue on physicians well-being.

Myers MF. Treatment of the mentally ill physician. Ottawa: Canadian Psychiatric Association; 2001.

Articles

Keim S et al Measuring wellness among resident physicians *Med Teach* 2006; 28(4):370-4.

Kaufmann M. Recognition and management of the behaviourally disruptive doctor. Ontario Medical Review 2001; 53-5 April.

Kaufmann M. Physician Suicide: risk factors and prevention. *Ont Med Rev* 2000; Sept 20-22

Glossary

Acronym	Term	Description
360°	360-degree evaluation aka Multi-source feedback	Direct reports, peers and supervisors complete forms to gather information, appraise conduct and provide feedback.
	Competencies	Used in the educational literature to refer to abilities, made up of knowledge, skills, and attitudes, that are essential for an individual to attain a larger competency.
	Constructed response format	A type of written test that asks learners to formulate their answers rather then to select the correct responses from a series of provided options.
CUSUM	Cumulative summary	Is a statistical technique that allows measurement of progress towards mastery of procedural skills by incorporating such components as adverse outcomes and frequency of repetition.
DEC	Daily encounter cards or daily evaluation cards	A type of in-training assessment tool characterized by observations that are documented after brief encounters between supervisor and learner in the clinical setting.
	Direct observation	In the Royal College model of in-training evaluation, direct observation refers to the ongoing observation, assessment and documentation of actions taken by the learners in real clinical settings during their training period. The critical factor that distinguishes direct observation from other forms of assessment is that the learner is observed performing authentic actions that occur naturally as part of the learner's daily clinical experience. As with simulation, direct observation requires the use of an associated assessment tool to structure and record the observer's judgment.

Acronym	Term	Description
DOC	Daily operative cards	A type of in-training direct observation characterized by observations that are documented after brief encounters between supervisor and learner in the clinical setting, in this case the operating room.
DTEC	Daily teaching evaluation cards	A type of teacher assessment tool characterized by observations that are documented after brief encounters between supervisor and learner in the clinical setting.
EMQ	Extended matching question	A type of written test in which learners are given a list of ten to twenty items and are asked to match them to a series of corresponding responses. An item may be matched to more than one response.
	Essays	A type of written test in which questions are asked that require the learners to construct an answer based on their knowledge in a written or computer-based format. Essays require the communication and synthesis of content and often require critical thinking skills such as evaluation, analysis and judgment.
	Extended matching	A type of written test in which learners are given a list of ten to twenty items and are asked to match them to a series of corresponding responses. An item may be matched to more than one response. For example, learners are given a list of organs and a list of drugs. Learners are asked to match the listed organs to the drugs that affect that organ.
	Fidelity	The degree of realism or authenticity of the assessment. For example, testing suturing skills on a pig has higher fidelity than surgical tubing.
FITER	Final In-Training Evaluation Report	A summative report on in-training assessment.

Acronym	Term	Description
	Halo effect	Is the positive influence upon scoring of all sub-items based on the perceived overall score—a positive skew. For example, a perceived outstanding learner will be given outstanding scores on all sub-items without specific regard to the learner's ability on the particular item. It is the opposite of the millstone effect.
ITER	In-Training Evaluation Report	An assessment instrument to document direct observation.
	Logbook	A structure instrument for documenting that a learning activity took place.
	Matching	A type of written test where learners are given two lists and are asked to match the items in one column to an item in the other column. As a common example, a list of terms in one column is matched with a list of their definitions in the other column.
	Millstone effect	The negative influence upon scoring of all sub-items based on the perceive overall score—a negative skew. For example, a perceived poor learner will be given poor scores on all sub-items without specific regard to the learner's ability on the particular item. It is the opposite of the halo effect.
MSF	Multi-source Feedback aka 360° feedback	A method that utilizes specific instruments, designed to gather data about specific behaviors or professional constructs (e.g., professionalism, communication skills) of the learner. A self assessment is frequently included. The questionnaires may be the same or different for each of the assessor groups. Feedback is provided in aggregate form for each source. MSF can be used to provide formative and summative assessments, and identify an individual in difficulty.
MCQ	Multiple-choice question	A type of written test that uses an opening question or *stem* that ask the learner to choose the most correct answer from a list that also includes two to five plausible yet incorrect *distracters*.

Acronym	Term	Description
	Oral examinations	An assessment method that involves an assessor or panel of assessors to pose a series of questions to a learner in order to assess and react to the learner's responses. Oral examinations allow a high level of dynamic assessor/learner interaction.
OSATS	Objective Structured Assessment of Technical Skills	Similar to an OSCE (see definition for *OSCE*), but focuses on psychomotor skills.
OSCE	Objective Structured Clinical Examinations	An assessment format that samples performance of learners as they rotate through a series of stations containing different clinical scenarios. At each station, learners may encounter a standardized patient, a structured oral, visual stimuli (e.g. X-rays, ECGs), a high or low fidelity simulation (e.g. part-task trainer), or a written task. Learners are usually asked to perform a specific skill, simulate part of a patient encounter or answer questions based on presented material.
OSPRE	Objective Structured Performance-Related Examination	Similar to an OSCE (see definition for *OSCE*), but does not necessarily have a clinical focus.
	Pick N	A type of written test where an amalgam of MCQ and extended matching, pick N items consist of an opening stem and an instruction to select any given number of correct responses from an extensive list. These questions may ask for all diagnostic tests or management actions that would be appropriate in a given clinical situation.
	Portfolios	A flexible, multifaceted method for collecting evidence of achievement of competence over time.
	Recall bias	A bias arising from mistakes in recollecting events, both because of failures of memory, and looking at things "with hindsight" and possibly changed views.

Acronym	Term	Description
	Selected response format	A type of written test that consists of a question and a list of options from which the learner must choose the correct answer. All selected response formats ask the learner to *recognize* the correct answer rather than recall it from memory without prompting. Multiple-choice, matching, extended matching, pick N and true/false questions are common tools within this category.
SAQ	Short-answer question	A type of written test that consists of a brief, highly directed question designed to elicit a reliable constructed response from the learner. Answers usually consist of a few short words or phrases. The model answer key is designed to comprehensively anticipate all correct answers.
	Simulated patients	Healthy actors trained to simulate a medical situation or condition.
	Simulation	The artificial re-creation of a clinical environment or circumstance for the purpose of allowing a learner to undertake a specific task in a controlled and patient-safe manner.
	Standardized patients	Can be either actual patients or healthy actors trained to simulate a medical situation or condition.
SOE	Structured oral examinations	An assessment method that assesses a set number of standardized cases using anticipated probing questions based on the range of expected candidate performance and anchored rating schemata to increase the reliability of the evaluation.
TEC	Teaching encounter cards	A type of in-training direct observation characterized by observations that are documented after brief encounters between supervisor and learner in the clinical setting.
	True–False	Learners are asked to determine if a given statement is true or false.

Made in United States
Cleveland, OH
05 November 2026

47664030R00063